The Art of Radical Self-Love

"*The Art of Radical Self-Love* is a wonderfully helpful book. Mary Joosten Lopata encouraged me to realize the great importance of how self-care enables us to learn compassion, forgiveness, and gratitude. I was struck by her beautiful phrasing and her conversational style and exercises for breathing."

ELIZABETH E. MCADAMS, PH.D.

"It was a joy reading *The Art of Radical Self-Love*. I found it not to be so much a read-it-and-put-it-on-the-shelf book but something I plan to review and implement again and again as my circumstances dictate. It's an informative reference, a primer, a guide, and an instructive "how to" manual. Mary provides both common sense reminders and many new paths to explore. This will most definitely be on my gift-giving list!"

KAREN MUSCARIELLO, HOSPICE & PALLIATIVE SERVICES

The Art of
Radical Self-Love

The First Steps to Healing & Well-Being

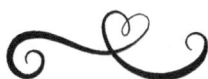

Mary Joosten Lopata, MA, RN

DeVorss Publications
Camarillo, California

The Art of Radical Self-Love

The information contained in this book, including ideas, theories, suggestions, exercises, and other materials, is provided as general information and is solely intended for the readers' own self-improvement and personal growth, to help in their quest for healing of mind, body, and spirit. The author and publishers of this book do not recommend nor prescribe the use of any technique as a form of treatment for medical or physical problems without the advice of a physician. It is not meant to be a substitute for medical or psychological treatment and does not replace the services of health-care professionals. If you experience emotional distress or physical discomfort using any of the ideas, theories, suggestions, or exercises in this book, you are advised to stop and seek professional care if appropriate.

Library of Congress Catalog Number: 2024003441
First DeVorss Publications Edition, 2024
Print ISBN: 9780875168538
Ebook ISBN: 9780875169545

DeVorss & Company, Publisher
PO Box 1389
Camarillo CA 93012
editorial@devorss.com

Printed in the United States of America
For more information, please visit www.devorss.com

Library of Congress Cataloging-in-Publication Data

Names: Lopata, Mary Joosten, author.
Title: The art of radical self-love : the first steps to healing & well-being / Mary Joosten Lopata, MA, RN.
Description: First DeVorss Publications edition. | Camarillo, California : DeVorss Publications, [2024] | Includes bibliographical references. | Summary: "The Art of Radical Self-Love IS A ROADMAP TO RESTORING PERSONAL WELLNESS FROM WITHIN. Includes a dynamic range of self-empowerment tools that nourish the journey to wellness. This guide treats healing as it truly is, an "art" that flows with the patient as needs fluctuate and shift to the ever-changing circumstances despite today's corporate-dictated healthcare system"—Provided by publisher. Identifiers: LCCN 2024003441 (print) | LCCN 2024003442 (ebook) | ISBN 9780875169538 (trade paperback) | ISBN 9780875169545 (ebook) Subjects: LCSH: Self-care, Health. | Mind and body therapies. | Healing. Classification: LCC RA776.95 .L667 2024 (print) | LCC RA776.95 (ebook) | DDC 613--dc23/ eng/20240301 LC record available at https://lccn.loc.gov/2024003441 LC ebook record available at https://lccn.loc.gov/2024003442

For my Mom,
who made my journey possible.

Acknowledgments

The author is deeply grateful for the support and encouragement from family, friends, clients, students, and healthcare colleagues who inspired this book.

The list is so long that I might inadvertently leave someone off of it, so I will trust that you know who you are. Thank you. Thank you. Thank you.

"Love is the crowning grace of humanity, the holiest right of the soul, the golden link which binds us to duty and truth, the redeeming principle that chiefly reconciles the heart to life, and is prophetic of eternal good."

—PETRARCH

Contents

"Experience is the hardest kind of teacher.
It gives you the test first and the
lesson afterward."

—OSCAR WILDE

Preface

There's a saying that if you respect your readers enough to tell your story honestly, you respect them enough to let them draw their own conclusions. I do not profess to be anywhere close to a perfected human being in my physical expression. At first I had misgivings about sharing my healing experiences, because what worked for me may not work for others in similar medical circumstances. That's the unknown nature of self-healing.

It is often said, we are all storytellers, and this is my story. I confess it was not an experiment I performed under a microscope of empirical science, where the results would be repeatable by others following my steps. And I am fairly certain no remedies I offer in this book will harm anyone—they may even greatly enhance wellness for some.

The invaluable life lessons I was taught during my cancer diagnosis motivated me to write this book, to share the health-giving tools and techniques I learned for my own therapeutic journey and which added to the empowering knowledge I gathered during the course of a lifetime of diligent study and practice as a holistic nurse. I pursued a registered nursing degree during the height of the HIV/AIDS epidemic and concurrent nursing shortage. I was recruited away from bedside postpartum nursing almost immediately by a third-party administrator for self-insured employers.

In the subsequent decades, with a variety of employers, I became a Certified RN Case Manager, a Certified Hospice and Palliative Care Nurse, a Certified Diabetic Educator, and a Board-Certified Holistic Nurse. I spent my professional career advocating for, coaching, and educating patients and their families regarding self-care and dealing with the broken health-care system, both as an employee and independent consultant.

My intention is to convey through the story of my healing journey, how I came to this curative approach, how the techniques shaped my life experiences, how you can fully embrace the restorative techniques I did when it came to your own healing miracle, and that there is a universal truth when you focus your energy on self-love and healing. My life's philosophy is that the underlying power of unconditional love is the common thread tying together all aspects of life. That's a hard statement to write; to some, it sounds simplistic and woo-woo, but so be it.

The beginning of this disconcerting yet illuminating odyssey can be traced back to a spring night in 2017, when I was struggling through a sleepless night. The pain in the right side of my abdominal area caused me to toss and turn, changing positions to see if the pain would stop. I knew my physical body well, and this was a persistent signal that needed attention. I got up and paced the floor to see if this would help ease the pain. For years, I had experienced other dramatic digestive symptoms that I often chose to ignore, which did indeed eventually go away. Although the discomfort was not intolerable—only annoying and continuous—I became concerned because the pain was not going away. I knew on a deeper level that something was seriously wrong and I needed to get the medical establishment involved. This did not make me happy.

I was disappointed in myself, as a holistic nurse of 30 years. Holistic nursing is a medical profession where nurses are dedicated to offering whole-person care to patients in need. Rather than treating a specific issue, holistic nurses look at the patient from a different perspective and examine their lifestyle for hints on how to improve their overall health and wellness. Whole-person nursing practice and integrative focus into other areas are key in holistic nursing. I held myself to be a teacher by example. I knew firsthand the benefits of living a healthy and empowered lifestyle. With certainty, I believed that emotions and thoughts influenced the physical body. I had read, learned from others, and experienced this health-affirming connection to myself. However, even teachers with an abundance of knowledge can, at times, get offtrack and allow themselves to go down a rabbit hole of negativity. If a problem is left unaddressed for a long enough time, mechanical damage can be done that requires outside professional care in order to fix the problem.

What caused my disappointment about this particular medical challenge was that I knew better than to let it happen to me, yet I felt I had unknowingly let it manifest in my body by not paying attention. I, who considered catching a cold to be a clarion call for self-renewal, had unconsciously wallowed in anger and resentment like a pig in mud for several years. The positive side of this self-healing philosophy was, I believed, if I got myself into this predicament, I could get myself out. But I knew this was a serious case, and I'd obviously need help. To quote the poet John Donne, "No man is an island entire of itself," which meant to me, "Here comes yet another lesson in humility. Oh, joy."

Over the years, I've seen firsthand with patients that abdominal pain is notoriously difficult to diagnose. My case was no different. The testing in the emergency department I visited that early morning in 2017 revealed two abnormalities, neither of which was ultimately the culprit. One was of little concern and merely became a footnote in my medical history. The most significant finding was a diseased gallbladder, and then the real snowball effect began. The gallbladder is the low hanging fruit of the diagnostic tree. After much reluctance and debate—months of me resisting intervention and writhing in pain—I reluctantly consented to allowing the diseased organ to be surgically removed that September.

I knew perhaps there would be postoperative symptoms. After all, the gallbladder is an important—although not essential—organ, and the sudden trauma of not having one can stress an already stressed digestive system. I then became tolerant of symptoms that I blamed on the aftereffects of surgery, especially recurring indigestion, and carried on as best I could. Of course, these postoperative symptoms are supposed to go away in a few months. After a year, I still had them. I'd allowed my attention to be redirected by various life tasks, such as moving into a new home and integrating myself into a new community once again. Then one night, 18 months later, I shot up in bed with crushing chest pain. I quietly slipped out of bed so as to not wake my husband, who was sleeping soundly. I somehow stumbled into the darkened bathroom, located the medicine cabinet and the bottle of Gaviscon, chewed up a couple of antacid tablets, drank some water, and paced around for what seemed like an eternity, fighting off panic and having an in-depth conversation with God or whatever other available, benevolent, invisible force of healing would listen to me. The pain passed after a couple of hours; exhausted, I finally went back to sleep.

The next day I went to see my husband's cardiologist. He did some testing that satisfied him that my heart was not in imminent danger and suggested I see a GI doctor. The medical term for this episode is a fart attack (as opposed to a heart attack), but only an ECG shows for sure. Well, she did what any good GI doc would do and soon I had tubes with cameras inserted to and fro within my body's digestive orifices. Fro was fine, but the other one showed a huge (her precise clinical description) polyp in my stomach that she was not comfortable removing at her outpatient surgery center. She referred me to a hospital-based GI surgeon she had met once at a social gathering hosted by the hospital for physicians to meet each other.

Here's where it got tricky. The surgeon I was first referred to was tasked with putting a scope into my stomach once again for the purpose of removing the polyp. I became concerned when I realized this surgeon was not a happy camper as I was waiting to go into the OR. I overheard her loud hallway conversations, complaining that she evidently was behind on her cases and in a hurry. So much so that she personally wheeled my bed into the OR in somewhat of a fury, banging it into walls on the way.

When I regained consciousness in the recovery room, the nurses told me the surgeon was not available to discuss what happened with me because she was performing another surgery. The nurses were apologetic, and I was uncomfortable because the procedure was so brief and I didn't have a urinary catheter. I was still wearing my own underwear with a bladder leak protection pad, which had soaked through without anyone else noticing. My husband, a type 2 diabetic, was at my bedside and impatient because neither of us had eaten for quite a while. I just wanted to go home, so the nurses arranged for me to be discharged, instructing me to make a follow-up appointment with the surgeon in her office.

I finally found out the details of my surgery at the post-op visit a couple weeks later. She told me she was only able to remove half of the polyp and sent it for a biopsy. She said she could go in again and try to get the rest of the polyp or do a wedge resection of my stomach. I asked for image copies of the endoscopy, and she gave me totally useless, indecipherable faxed copies and said that was the best she could provide.

When the biopsy results came in, they were "concerning." I was referred to another GI surgeon, this one a professor at a prodigious medical school. Perhaps this would be better. My initial consultation had her fellow physician learning the specialty present as well. I had a sinking feeling that it was not a good thing for my case to be considered a teaching opportunity—I was right. The pathology results mentioned "rare and scattered neuroendocrine cells," from a biopsy that this new surgeon described as "aggressive."

When speaking with a surgeon before having an operation, no one ever wants to hear, "You need to have a further workup beforehand so we can see if it has metastasized." I was shocked to hear that I now had the misfortune of a diagnosis of a neuroendocrine tumor of the stomach. It used to be called a "carcinoid" tumor, which basically means slow-growing cancer that could progress into full-blown cancer if you live long enough. Notice, my "polyp" had been replaced by "tumor," and if it had metastasized, this potentially new diagnosis offered no treatment options or hope and was considered terminal.

"It ain't what you don't know that gets you in trouble. It's what you know for sure that just ain't so."

—ANONYMOUS

Introduction

I, like the many other cancer patients I have nursed over the last three decades, was stunned at that dreaded moment on May 30, 2019, when the doctor's shocking diagnosis pushed me onto the cancer treatment roller-coaster ride.

All my life I have had a love/hate relationship with roller coasters. Sometimes they're fun. Sometimes they're terrifying. It quickly became clear this would not be an enjoyable experience. That arduous ride lasted until October 30, 2019—five solid months of daily, intensely focused behavior modification and radical self-love with the hope I would someday safely exit the ride. Visiting the cancer center at the hospital for testing and consults was scary, to say the least. The building itself has someone's name in giant lettering and "Memorial" on it, indicating that even an extremely wealthy person probably wasn't cured, despite such heroic interventions.

The weeks of testing were grueling, both physically and psychologically, and seemed endless. Every time I entered the building I felt like I was ringside at an arena where doom and hope battled each other, with uncertainty acting as referee.

I don't want to relive that free-floating anxiety. I had been there every step during my late husband's colon cancer journey as we visited similar clinics; now I was on the patient side of the medical experience, and it was positively overwhelming. At times I felt powerless, even with my extensive knowledge of both personal and professional backstories. Suffice to say, I gained a layer of compassion and understanding for cancer patients that will never be lost. It was a difficult time because I was so encapsulated in my challenging healing experience, I had little energy to share with my current husband or children, to ask how they were feeling about this situation. I realized, at times like this, healing does have to be all about you. It's okay to give yourself permission to invest all your time and energy into just taking loving care of yourself.

I understand how hard it is to become your own self-healing advocate, especially after getting bad news. Surgeon #2's treatment plan was to remove the lower half of my stomach, including the valve that connects it to my small intestine, along with a portion of the intestine. Then they would sew the intestine back to what was left of my stomach. That kind of sounded like I would need to eat while sitting on the toilet for the rest of my life. No, thank you. After extensive research, I explored alternatives to the working diagnosis. This was not magical thinking. A diagnosis is only a physician's name for what they theorize your problem is based on the data they have. Doctors are taught to make a diagnosis and never waver from it unless future empirical data completely contradicts it; even then, they may cling to their original thought pattern.

It is a very empowering decision to say "No, thank you" to your treating physician's diagnosis and treatment plan.

By law, only licensed physicians are allowed to diagnose and definitively declare they know what's wrong with you and what they think should be done about it. I doubted the conclusions being drawn by the doctor and the treatment plan that proceeded from them, and therefore formed my own alternative explanation based on my education and experience. I do not advise this practice for most patients because, as I already revealed, I can be a contrarian when it comes to my personal health-care decisions. However, I do advise getting an unbiased second surgical opinion when major body parts are going to be removed or rearranged and it's not an immediate life-threatening emergency.

My alternative diagnostic theory was that the rare, scattered neuroendocrine cells found in the biopsy specimen of the polyp originated from the tissue in the stomach, where they naturally occur and which had been included in the polyp tissue. When I was given this diagnosis, I was frankly embarrassed. I had been a holistic wellness nurse-coach who had obviously not been practicing what she preached. I heeded the wake-up call. I took a shotgun approach to my action plan, and I returned to loving myself enough to ask for help and do my part. I prayed, meditated, focused on a positive outcome, apologized to my body for doing this to it, forgave myself for behaviors that led to this problem, did affirmations, joined a daily healing circle, and accepted any and all offers of prayers and spiritual/energetic assistance. I modified my diet and took USP-tested vitamins and supplements.

I got out and walked in nature as best I could. And I had all the prescribed medical testing done and kept my doctors' appointments. I created a sort of eight-step holistic healing program for myself that combined health care and the humanities, which I've distilled into the chapters of this book. I committed to being an active daily participant in my health and well-being, and kept track of my progress. I decided I was worth the extra effort it would take to change my behaviors, and I began each day with an energy treatment for myself. I used breathwork throughout the day to energize, calm, relax, and balance my emotions and also as a gateway to meditation. I recited affirmations throughout the day to motivate me to act on my intentions to manifest love, health, forgiveness, and gratitude. I found something to laugh about every day, and I followed a nutrition plan for clean eating, took some supplements, and got daily exercise as well as adequate sleep. I even involved my family and friends for support in my journey.

After my wake-up call, I asked if Surgeon #2 could remove the remainder of the polyp and see what it held before going any further. I thought I was clear about this course of action until I was actually in the OR, where she informed me that she was going to have her fellow take a look-see into my stomach to stage prior to my future partial stomach and intestine removal. I protested. I told her our agreement was that she would personally do the case and she would remove the remainder of the polyp for biopsy, after which we would discuss further treatment. Which I discovered she did after I woke up in the recovery room. The final pathology results? Inflamed polyp, no signs of cancer. Our post-op visit was special. She did have the good grace to thank me for pushing her in the right direction.

The unanswered question remains: Was it a miracle or a misdiagnosis?

The medical establishment had data to support a cancer diagnosis and the rationale for radical surgical intervention. However, after numerous months-long, unexplainable delays in scheduling and a last-minute change in the mind of the surgeon in the OR, the outcome was completely different from what was medically anticipated in the beginning. Was it a miracle that the misdiagnosis was found before half my stomach and part of my intestine was removed? Or was the miracle that there was no error in diagnosis at the onset, but through the interventions of love, prayer, and positive energy and actions, the body reverted to its undiseased state? The obstructing polyp, of course, had to go, but it was formed as a defensive reaction to an irritant that had just gone wild.

To me, it doesn't matter. It was a warning for me to become self-responsible for what my body needed. My stomach is intact, and I affirm every day that I am healthy and cancer-free. Some people don't like to use the word *cancer* but I'm not afraid of it. I am in a proactive, preventative health-care lifestyle. My takeaway is that we must be actively constructive in our thoughts and actions, not merely passive, so that letting Nature take its course is for our continued health and wellness. Nature's expression can be influenced by our intentions. Intending a most benevolent outcome for our highest and best good is a comforting affirmation to live by.

In this book, I share how our bodies are amazing, unique biological expressions of physical, mental, and spiritual experiences that we don't completely understand because we don't yet comprehend how to integrate all the input to produce the desired outcome of a comfortable lifespan. According to Florence Nightingale, the founder of modern nursing, medicine's use is to remove an obstruction to cure, and nursing's job is to put the patient in the best condition for nature to affect a cure. I'm good with that

I cannot definitively claim that I experienced a miracle. In my heart, I know I did, so the opinions of others are irrelevant. I know what the diagnosis was according to pathology in the beginning, and I know what the diagnosis was at the end based on pathology. Doubters can say that initially it must have been a misdiagnosis. Doesn't matter. Right now, I'm well. Perhaps I experienced spontaneous remission (or spontaneous regression, a variation on the same thing), which is a clinically acceptable term for a miracle. There are things in common that those who are considered to have experienced spontaneous remission changed in their lives. I intuitively dipped into the wellspring they used for guidance and wisdom to make changes in mine. Depending on the researcher, there are around 10 factors that folks applied to their lives that favored the disappearance of disease. I chose the behaviors that I felt I would consistently practice.

Reflecting on my path to recovery, I realized I had followed much of what the Institute of Noetic Sciences' researchers' studies on spontaneous remission of cancer had documented. It was evidently stored in the recesses of my nurse-coach memory banks in case an opportunity arose, thank goodness.

As my health challenges concluded, I was inspired by a feeling of responsibility to spread my revelations further than a few close friends. When you get to my age, if you've got something to say, it's time to say it. So I put together an outline of the healing path I took on my journey to serve as a quick reference, to remind whoever reads it that we have control over our mind and imagination. By creatively using that talent we have the ability to change unhealthy behaviors and change the course of our lives. Think of it like a healing cookbook with a collection of personal recipes that use easily available ingredients that most are familiar with but may not be using to their highest potential.

Afterwards, I began writing the key points of my recovery guide for a class I was scheduled to teach in person for eight weeks, beginning on March 15, 2020. I had prepared class outlines for the teaching modules, which are more extemporaneous in design than a text. The individual classes were scheduled to be about an hour and a half each, once a week, for eight weeks, and since I consider my signed-up attendees to be peers well-versed in the subject matter, I expected productive feedback within the learning framework that would benefit both them and me and which would adequately fill in the class time allowed.

At the time of writing this book, I had no social media platform, published books, podcasts, or blogs. I am, however, a retired Certified Holistic Registered Nurse, which means love and spirituality are the foundation of my healing philosophy. What I have to offer is the knowledge and experience of a lifetime of researching and personally applying health theories that are both mainstream and metaphysical. There is a lot of evidence that alternative and complementary health-care treatments are effective. After years of teaching and accepting this, I had the opportunity to put it into action in my own life and proved its truth to my satisfaction. My hope is that you will benefit from my lessons and see that if I can do it, so can you.

That initial class didn't happen because of the initial COVID-19 pandemic isolation rules. As the months went by, it occurred to me that other people might benefit from a health and wellness self-reliance plan. I committed to a project: sharing tools to rekindle healing and love on a personal level that would then spread globally.

My intention is to offer self-healing wisdom that others may be inspired to put into practical use. What I'm sharing is my take on what worked for me, because I certainly cannot try out every theory that comes down the health-care highway. I have attempted to strike a balance in blending empirical science and complementary and/or alternative paths. My personal bias is toward a holistic approach which is inclusionary, using whatever works.

The basis of these lifestyle changes is taking action in your own life. I'm not suggesting that you shouldn't get conventional medical treatment when an injury or disease disrupts your physical health. I'm also not suggesting that you stop there. We're best served having a holistic approach to restoring and maintaining our health. My medical treatment plan included taking supplements and vitamins, as well as seriously changing my diet. It also involved surgery and a lot of annoying diagnostic tests. Conventional medicine had nothing else to offer, so I added complementary approaches to that mix.

I am not an authority on your body. Besides my personal experiences, I do have access to a treasure trove of other people's reported successful healing experiences by virtue of being a nurse, Reiki master, hypnotherapist, and independent researcher. I'm choosing to share what I feel are the best gems to start or add to your personal treasure chest of valuable health and wellness practices. Please feel free to expand your personal collection from the basics I'm offering.

This book is organized with stand-alone chapters, so there's a bit of repetition, especially with breathing exercises and journaling. Each chapter has educational information, a personal story about applying the information, and practical exercises to integrate it into your life. By the way, I already knew all of this when I began my intense healing journey—knowing and doing are two different things. The information was scattered in different sources, including my imperfect memory. I wrote the handbook I wish I'd had, with all the pertinent information in one place. I want it to be practical, informative, and useful.

My medical records still contain the diagnosis "malignant neoplasm of the stomach," even though the final pathology report states "no cancer detected." The past is not erased, but rather stands for me as a reminder of the power of choice.

In closing, to paraphrase the Buddhist monk Thich Nhat Hanh, "I realize that I cannot infuse anyone else with healing wisdom. I can only encourage you to recognize it is already inside you and to wake it up and allow it to guide you as you desire." I am grateful for the gift of that frightening journey, because there is nothing like firsthand experience to teach compassion—for yourself and others.

The Art of Radical Self-Love

MARY JOOSTEN LOPATA

"You already have the precious mixture
that will make you well. Use it."

—RUMI

CHAPTER ONE

The Healing Journey

Setting Your Healing Intentions and
Engaging Your Own Consciousness

THE FUNDAMENTAL PHILOSOPHY of radical loving self-care is holistic healing–body, mind, and spirit–all deciding for life in balance and cooperation. Being proactive by choosing sacred selfishness is a radical decision for self-care.

When I received the cancer diagnosis that spurred me to return to taking self-directed healing actions, I was stunned. I thought I'd established a healthy lifestyle pattern that would make me virtually invincible to disease. Really, I was that cocky. It was now clear I'd become complacent in my daily practices and was living my life as if I knew nothing about the healing power of holistically maintaining my health and well-being. I mean, if you want to know the truth, look at the results.

Just having knowledge is useless without application. I learned after my own diagnosis how an effective path to healing means going back to consistent self-love practices that provide access to an empowering source of one's own ability to heal the mind and body. My intention as a nurse and holistic teacher is to assist you in finding your own personal healing path in the garden of your life and caring for it at whatever level you desire right now.

What exactly is healing?

The word "healing" has a lot of meanings. My accepted holistic health definition is that healing is the ongoing process of bringing all aspects of your body/mind/spirit into balance at deeper levels of inner knowing. Healing involves the coordination and cooperation of all our moving parts, seen and unseen. Healing is coming home to ourselves. Healing is not necessarily curing, although curing involves healing. The outcome of your healing work results from your personal path's intention. Be gentle and gracious with yourself when encountering the wisdom of not knowing everything.

In this book, I offer experiences based on the many different teachings on the art and science of healing. The art portion comes from the creative unconscious reality and the science part comes from the rational reality. In nursing, we say that you can teach anyone how a machine works, but you can't teach anyone how to care. To bring about lasting healing, we must care. For our purposes, we must care deeply about ourselves and our highest and best good, because that's all we have control over.

As caring, conscious beings, we are living as guests on a planet that is often sorely out of balance. I believe we must all do our part and are tasked with loving the world back to health, one person at a time. This healing must begin with ourselves. I realize that's a little heavy, but I wanted to introduce my philosophy that the *big picture* concept gives meaning to the whole exercise and continuously runs in the background. My interpretation of this picture is a very simplified version of a theory of everything that works for me—briefly, this short time we live on Earth is not all there is, and we're all in this together.

Healing takes time. But not healing also takes time. It's the same amount of a finite commodity. How you spend it is a personal choice. Do you want to spend your time healing or not healing? There are as many paths to healing as there are individuals. It is exquisitely personal. In my research, healing is associated with belief. I believe that both love and fear require a belief in something invisible, but they are mutually exclusive; one cannot exist in the presence of the other. It is our choice which of them we take as our guiding principle.

Fear is a great motivator for human beings. It comes directly from our primal animal instinct to survive. We need to determine the difference between concrete fear—when something is immediately going to physically harm us—and baseless fears like the fear of missing out, which are just going to make us psychologically uncomfortable. Our reptilian brain does not differentiate between the two. If we are not in mortal danger, we need to examine where the fear is coming from so we can take our power back. What belief of ours is causing the same reaction as though we're about to die?

There is a common problematic pattern in all belief systems. The problem is not about learning; it is about integrating the lessons learned into our daily lives. We can use an acronym for illusionary fear to deal with it: **F**ace it, **E**xamine it, **A**ccept it, **R**everse it. (Another is **F**alse **E**vidence **A**ppearing **R**eal.) We need to recognize emotional fear, which is based on beliefs that no longer serve us, and establish the habit of replacing it with love.

What or who is directing the belief does not matter. One can believe completely in contemporary Western medicine, or traditional Chinese medicine, or alternative medicine, or folkloric medicine, or faith healing, or any combination of those, along with other beliefs. Healing has been taking place before there was any organized approach to it. Healing often seems to be a mystery that may or may not be apparent to an observer or participant. It doesn't matter. Healing happens. Some interventions appear to facilitate healing. That's what this book will explore.

This book's purpose, as I see it, is to provide tools for you to integrate the lessons physically, mentally, and spiritually.

Trauma creates the need for healing. Not only is trauma stored as memories in our minds and spirits, but our bodies also have a consciousness that is capable of storing trauma. It would follow then that for permanent healing, we need to address all three levels and keep them connected and communicating on good terms with one another.

Conventional Western medicine is pretty much limited to combining the physical and mental, generally leaving the spiritual component to religion. Religion sometimes connects the spiritual and mental in hopes of positively affecting the physical. Integrated medicine is trending toward addressing all three, but only if there is reimbursement possible through evidence-based standards of practice. (Oops, that's my bias showing.) Psychosomatic medicine studies the relationship of social, psychological, and behavioral factors on how physical bodies respond to them. Holistic health care, meanwhile, is unabashedly based on the healing properties of unconditional love; if science can quantify that energy and information, wonderful. Until then, we'll carry on until they catch up.

There are a multitude of holistic health modalities about which I have just a smattering of knowledge, like tapping (EFT, an alternative treatment for physical pain and emotional distress). HeartMath taps into the power and intelligence of your heart—your heart's intuition—which awakens you to the best version of yourself. Neuro-linguistic programming (NLP, a pseudoscientific approach to communication, personal development, and psychotherapy), crystals, aroma-therapy, essential oils, bodywork, muscle testing, etc. all offer different methods of reaching the source of our ailments. This work will just address areas where I believe I can provide useful, effective life practices in a short period of time, based on my personal experience, education, and practice. It is not all-encompassing. I honor the knowledge of others, but we must stay on point because I don't know everything—and I never will, but I'm still very curious. I'm okay with that, and I hope you are, too.

Truth does not care about our beliefs. If science shows conclusively that our beliefs are wrong, we need to change our beliefs. The Earth is not flat. Healing should not be a competition between belief systems, but rather a flexible, cooperative application of what works for the individual. We need to keep an open mind with a critical filter. In my specific case, the large growth in my stomach was real and needed to be surgically removed. On the other hand, there was a glitch in how my stomach cells reproduced that allowed the growth to form. That's the unseen cause. Holistic healing is about addressing the underlying cause, seen or unseen.

We are all on this journey together. I have been a healing coach and a nurse facilitator over the last 30 years, but I am not a saint. A saint, as I understand it, is a perfected human being. Although I strive to practice what I preach, I am fully human and imperfect. We have "best" practices because there are also "good" and "better." Please do not let perfection get in the way of good. We are together on a continuum that flows back and forth from seeker to wayfinder to wisdom keeper. Two steps forward and one step back is still net progress. Let's be determined yet gentle with ourselves.

My goal is to offer you understanding, not a definitive solution. People who appear to struggle are on the exact path they choose, and people are free to make their own choices. As the Dalai Lama said, "Just because they're not on your road, doesn't mean they're lost." My wish is that all of us allow the flow, understanding that the answer to our requests is not always what we would interpret as a "Yes." It may well be that we didn't get exactly what we asked for because we are being protected from some unforeseen secondary occurrence. The Chinese farmer parable about "Good Luck, Bad Luck, Who Knows?" comes to mind. Nothing is good or bad unless our judgment makes it so, and hindsight can change that opinion.

To prove to ourselves that our healing intentions are getting results, it's useful to keep track of what we are asking for, lest we forget and not notice all the little related experiences that happen. People call this asking and receiving process by many different names: mind treatment, prayer, affirmations, positive thinking, miracles, etc.

In health-care science, radical healing is sometimes called spontaneous—or unexpected—remission. For simplicity, we'll just call it keeping track of our requests. Our requests can be elaborate and well-thought-out or off the cuff and instantaneous. Doesn't matter what you're asking for. It could be anything from a parking space opening up to a good surgery outcome. You need to trust the process and write it down in a dated journal.

The first course of radical loving self-care requires a dated journal to track what is asked for and the results. Whether it's a digital notebook or good ol' pencil and paper, it's an important part of reinforcing successes, large and small. When we write our wishes down, it creates a concrete record of what we want and what we got. Sometimes my results are delightful and sometimes they're confusing. Nonetheless, journaling is a good way to integrate desired changes into our lives. This book is about radical loving self-care, so we can use the concepts for all areas of life that would benefit from healing by affirming our desired state or conditions.

Affirmations are verbal statements that direct your subconscious to the desired state of being. They are not to be confused with Star Trek's Captain Picard saying "Make it so," which implies the condition currently does not exist. The affirmation needs to state that it is so. You're telling your subconscious to manifest or maintain conditions in your life as if the desired condition already exists.

These verbal statements then restore the perfect energy in your subconscious that leads to growth and manifestation.

That is why many affirmations end with "And so it is." Perhaps in Star Trek "reality" Picard should have actually said, "It is so."

Affirmations are intensely personal and individual. At the end of each chapter, I'll provide some suggested affirmations that you can use as a starting point. Make each affirmation an "I am" statement in the present tense, form each one positively, and hold the intention that it is for your highest good. As you start, write them down and say them out loud. Revise them until they feel right, then memorize them to repeat whenever you need reminding.

Even though I don't know everything, like health and well-being teachers such as Oprah, I know some things for sure. Based on my professional experience as a holistic nurse, I know for sure that affirmations work. Just a word of caution: A radical self-love practice that directs your subconscious is only concerned with you. It is not taking into consideration that fulfilling your commands may also be creating unanticipated complications involving other people. So just tell your subconscious what you want the final result to be and don't insert how your rational mind (ego) thinks it should be done. Keep it simple. Keep it specific. For mental clarity in making formal requests, I find it helpful to center myself before journaling.

Affirmation Examples:

"I am thankful for my health, and I am
grateful for my health."

"I am clear and focused on my goals."

"I give thanks for the expression of infinite life,
health, and energy."

Healing Exercise:

Sit comfortably straight in a chair, feet flat on the floor. Consciously relax your body, and focus on your solar plexus, which is about two inches below your belly button, or focus on your heart space, whichever you choose. Set the intention that this self-directed activity is for your highest and best good. Breathe in through your nose, into your stomach area, and then up into your chest, then exhale through your mouth at whatever depth and rate is comfortable for you. Close your eyes, breathe, and relax into the intention to do what best serves you. As you breathe, feel the energy of unconditional love that always surrounds you and fills every cell. Breathe in and out a few more times, then open your eyes and begin journaling or whatever else you wanted to do. Once you get the hang of centering, you can do it anywhere, anytime. You won't need to necessarily sit and close your eyes. You'll remember how it feels when you're centered, and it will keep you from feeling scattered.

Write down in your request journal the central result you want fulfilled by reading this book. You can change it anytime you want, but it'll be interesting to see what you wanted at the beginning. Here are some prompting questions: Do you want to love and care for yourself differently? Do you want to heal something specific within yourself? Do you want to be more proactive in loving self-care? Do you want to decide for life? Do you want validation that in taking care of yourself with loving intention, you are helping to heal the world? Your wish, of course, can be totally different from these. Or you can wish I'd stop with the audience participation and just let you read already! No worries, it's just a suggestion.

Follow-Up Thoughts:

I would like to reiterate that healing is a continuum, which means it changes gradually while staying part of a whole concept whose beginning and ending points are very different from each other. Love is the key element in healing, and self-healing especially requires surrender to unconditional love by focusing on finding love, forgiveness, and gratitude in every moment.

Personally, I find this practice very challenging. Even during the solitude of my daily walk, when I've set the intention to keep repeating the word "love" as my mantra and block out all other thoughts, I often find myself repeating the catchy lyrics of a song that has the same rhythm as my pace without noticing right away that I've changed focus. I start remembering things I thought I'd forgiven and forgotten. Breathe deep, center, begin again. Healing grows and evolves just as love does, following our intentions. We cannot simply do nothing and expect the healing we desire to take place. We must intend healing and act toward that result. Symptoms of disease indicate a need for change, since the status quo is uncomfortable. We can only create in the now, so we focus on healing in the present tense, even if the demonstration of healing is not evident to our physical senses immediately.

Now, here's the buzzkill. Healing is not our golden ticket to physical immortality. Eventually, no matter how many times we are healed or how virtuously we live our lives, bodily death will occur. There's an awful lot of evidence that some type of afterlife exists and that it is a continuously love-filled environment compared to the emotional struggles on Earth. I'm okay with that assumption. So my position is that what we call death is nothing to be afraid of. What we term "bodily death" is a transition from one form of reality to another—a shift in consciousness. I've been to the brink and back, and this book is about taking care of ourselves the best we can while we're here so we can truly learn love, compassion, forgiveness, and gratitude and share them with others. That is the core of healing, and we teach best by example.

"If your compassion does not include yourself, it is incomplete."

—JACK KORNFIELD

CHAPTER TWO

Sacred Selfishness

Maintaining Awareness of Self-Love and
Confidence within Your Own Healing Power

K INDNESS IS A KEY ATTRIBUTE OF LOVE, and kindness
starts with being kind to yourself. Sacred selfishness
expands on that and establishes a priority of falling in love
with ourselves again. In our lives, it's easy to forget that at
the core of being is love, which is realizing we deserve kindness. It is the opposite of what we commonly define as selfishness. For many of us, the suggestion that being selfish is
a good thing is a radical concept. Sacred selfishness is a loving concern for one's own well-being. Our consciousness is
entitled to reverence and respect. Sacred selfishness is a holy
concept which rejects the idea of being separated. Instead,
it supports the underlying philosophy that all is connected,
but we only have a choice about our personal experiences.

Most likely, we have been raised to be "approval junkies,"
acting in ways that will benefit and please others but which are

not necessarily in alignment with our core values. Religious or societal teachings that conflict with our higher values are enforced, and we follow them because we are afraid. We think it's safer to be anonymous and infer agreement, but that internal conflict can cause stress and lead to sickness.

We need to unlearn the erroneous indoctrination that we are not worthy. Only then can we realize that pursuing the good of our higher selves is the goal of our lives. That goal will naturally include service to others, as long as it does not require a disservice to ourselves. In other words, it is up to us to unbreak our hearts.

The criterion for sacred selfishness is not looking to anyone else's judgment for approval. Your attention shifts to bring you more happiness, more life-affirming joy, more peace into yourself, and at the same time harms no one. There you have it.

The word "selfish" is generally burdened with a negative vibe for most of us. Being labeled selfish is not usually taken as a compliment. Early on, children are taught to share, often with the command, "Don't be selfish." We learn that being selfless is a desired character value in major religions, where the message can be interpreted that other people should be more valued than oneself. For example, in the Christian Bible, the commandment, "Love your neighbor as yourself," appears to imply that we have a healthy self-esteem that is to be reflected in our treatment of others.

Gautama Buddha reportedly said, "You must love yourself before you love another. By accepting yourself and fully being what you are, your simple presence can make others happy." We do no service to love our neighbor as ourselves if we don't love ourselves first. What would we have to offer if we are giving to others what we don't even give ourselves? Learning and practicing self-love can be the most difficult task in our healing journey. It requires an unwavering strength and commitment that will be well worth it.

The word "selfish" has more than one meaning, like most words do. Sure, it can mean the dreaded seeking only of one's own pleasure by destroying the comfort of others, thinking exclusively about the outcome for oneself, regardless of anyone else. On the other hand, good selfishness brings others, like family and friends, into the circle of prosperity as you prosper, rather like abundance profit sharing. Sacred selfishness goes one step further and recognizes that taking good care of oneself holistically will benefit humanity, because what one does for oneself will be positively expanded for the good of all.

There is a reason that airline safety drills instruct us to put the oxygen mask on ourselves before attempting to assist others. Unless we are able to live and breathe, we are not in the position to help anyone else do likewise.

Daily practice of sacred selfishness removes the feeling of "not being enough," because it empowers you. If you are not an advocate for yourself, who will be? Is someone else's happiness more important than your own? Can you forgive yourself for not being perfect by standards created by someone else? Others can teach and advise, but ultimately it is your decision and yours alone to see yourself as a deserving, independent, capable, and loving person. Personal responsibility is not blame—it is a natural by-product of free will. You alone own your life experience. How you choose to practice self-love is personal to you and only you know what your heart is telling you. It is your story.

We would do well to address and rid ourselves of the mental and emotional conditioning that comes from a culture steeped in the traditions of the zero-sum model of competition for resources. If we get something, it doesn't follow that someone else will be deprived of it. That contradicts basic supply and demand, doesn't it? If there's demand for something, the marketplace will supply it. You may be restrained from taking someone else's resources, but equivalent resources will be made available to you. Sacred selfishness has similarities to the popular "Law of Attraction" principle that you will attract into your life whatever you focus on.

The Law of Attraction has been popularized by accumulating material wealth, but abundance can be anything; in this case we want to attract an abundance of self-love for the purpose of self-healing. And if nothing else, I sincerely hope that after reading this book, you will have a balanced understanding of the true value of being able to use your energy to heal yourself as well as how to use it to accumulate things. Stuff is fun to have, but since you can't take it with you, it's hard to parlay that into a reason for living to heal yourself.

Remember, your past experiences were just lessons, not a life sentence which leaves you to repeat the same mistakes over and over again. Don't be discouraged at starting over. You're not starting from scratch—you're starting fresh with new experience. Begin each day anew with gratitude, resolution, and determination. You're worth every bit of effort you invest in becoming the most empowered and healthy version of you.

If you fail and try again, you won't remember the failure, but if you fail and don't try again, you'll remember the failure. No matter how much time your journey takes or how challenging a new behavior is to include in your daily practice, please stay true to your commitment to say "Yes!" to yourself.

Saying "Yes!" to ourselves sometimes requires us to say "No" to someone or something else. Saying "No" can feel risky, but we always have that right. Some of us may have been conditioned in childhood not to say "No." We need to remember to speak with our adult voices. We also have the mirror obligation to honor someone else saying "No" to us.

Once you can outline the problem in detail, then you will be able to see the solution. Set specific goals and deadlines. A goal is a dream with a deadline. Keep your word to yourself. When you set deadlines, it will help you to bring up matters that need to be done or discussed; therefore by all means, keep these commitments to yourself. If something is too difficult right now, modify your goal. It's your life and your story—you're allowed to change your mind. Your energy will naturally fluctuate in intensity. You don't need to force it. People are capable of accomplishing what they dream of at any time in their lives.

Here are some samples of radical loving self-care sacred selfishness affirmations to counter negative unconscious programming, which includes not feeling worthy, feeling responsible for others, and feeling that being spiritual requires total selflessness. Affirmations are good mental reminders to keep us in the present. Human nature has a tendency to backslide a little when everything feels okay and other things have our attention, especially in health-care matters. Feel free to write your own affirmations. Maybe you'd like to record them in your journal and check back and note the results.

Affirmation Examples:

"I am healing now. I am receiving healing forever and always."

"What's good and healthy for me is good and healthy for others."

"I am a loving and powerful caregiver to myself."

Healing Exercise:

Purse your lips like you're making a fish face, place the thumb and forefinger of your dominant hand on either side of your mouth, apply gentle pressure to make your lips part, and say "No." Relax and repeat two more times. You may want to do this in a mirror a few times to get the expression and timing down.

This may sound like a silly thing to do, but it may come in handy when someone is violating your boundaries. If you are a giver by nature, you must set limits because takers don't have any. Back in the day when I was PTA president at my children's school, the requests for volunteer hours kept going up, following the adage that if you want something done, ask a busy person to do it. Volunteering can present a slippery slope for approval junkies. So, we'd perform this little exercise at the beginning of the meeting and then proceed with business, sorting out inappropriate tasks. It was our own little "Just Say No" program.

You may enjoy a game of identifying examples of how you reinforce a nonpositive mindset just to heighten your awareness. For example, pay attention to how the media churns out never-ending, often conflicting, information about how to attain the preferred (by whom?) level of health and beauty, and therefore acceptance and admiration of others. Body image dissatisfaction has been hammered into us. We need to change the way we think about ourselves and become our own nonjudgmental best friend forever. A useful practice is to recognize that another's criticism of you is a reflection of what they're not happy about with themselves. It really has nothing to do with you. This is also true of your criticism of another. There's no need to judge—just allow yourself to become immune to negativity from any source, including yourself.

Every day, when you get up, stand in front of a mirror, put your hand over your heart, and smile. That's it! See yourself as worthy and enough, and carry that vision of yourself throughout the whole day.

Follow-Up Thoughts:

We are all a work in progress. Be gentle but persistent. The gifts of loving and caring that we truly need come from within ourselves and are condition-free. You deserve them just because you are unique—truly one of a kind.

There is an ancient Greek word, *philautia*, which is translated as self-love, meaning unconditional self-acceptance with empathy and appreciation for oneself. Aristotle reasoned that self-love can be either bad, when it is solely for personal gain, or the highest type of good, when it is exercised to promote virtue. That's basically the difference between prideful selfishness, which is a distortion of the good, and sacred selfishness, which is caring for and respecting oneself. It is healthy to make yourself a priority and act in your own best interests, as long as your intention is to cause no harm. We can take credit for our successes without demeaning anyone else or being boastful. It's just a matter of sticking to the observable results. Avoid self-blame, since that's an ego-based control issue. Make small realistic goals and look for solutions rather than problems. Be fearless in embracing your inner power and the whole game will change.

And then, we can breathe easier.

"If you want to find the secrets of the universe, think in terms of energy, frequency, and vibration."

—NIKOLA TESLA

CHAPTER THREE

Accessing Healing Energy

Inviting the Higher Life-Force Energy to
Guide You on Your Healing Journey

WE ARE ENERGY BEINGS. We live bathed in an ocean of energy. There are seemingly different kinds of fields of energy within us and all around us, natural and man-made, that we exchange, absorb, and are supported by. We are best served by being in the flow of the energetic fields that resonate with our highest good. We can name these good vibrations or beneficial frequencies. They are always present, but free will dictates that we request access to them.

Healing energy comes from a field that many experts call life-force energy. My holistic health belief is that the life force that animates the body heals the body. We can invite the life-force energy present in the universe to come into our bodies and spirits for the healing and promotion of health. This energy is infinitely abundant and available to everyone. What can happen as a person absorbs it is a feeling of relaxation and surrender that helps the body balance and heal itself.

Whether we call it the universal life-force energy, the Source, All That Is, One Mind, the frequency domain, the collective unconscious—or something else, like Truth, God, Universal Mind, or The Big Bang—it exists as unconditional love and awaits prompting and direction.

Science is studying the biophysical effects of energy, but not enthusiastically. Energy medicine, part of integrative medicine, is the use of known subtle energy fields to assess and treat energetic imbalances to bring the body's systems back to homeostasis, or balance. Specialties in holistic and energy medicine include hypnotherapy, healing touch, imagery, massage, meditation, Reiki, spiritual/transpersonal healing/prayer, therapeutic touch, traditional Chinese medicine, Emotional Freedom Techniques like tapping, HeartMath, and yoga/breathwork, just to name a few.

There are clinical studies correlating the overlap of the chakra system with the endocrine system and their associated electrical frequencies. The chakra system could have its own chapter, but in a nutshell, it is a theoretical arrangement of seven energy centers in the body, from the base of the spine to the top or crown of the head. Each center has its own color, vibration, or frequency and area of influence on the body. Merging metaphysics and physics, especially quantum physics, with biochemistry is an ongoing challenge.

I have this habit of attempting to quantify that which is possibly only qualitative. It's my holistic nursing background, where efforts are made to defend doing what works without fully understanding how or why it works. In other words, there are health practices considered folklore by empirical science that are nonetheless effective in real-life applications. Energy healing is one such practice. There's a lot of pushback from the very lucrative pharmaceutical industry—and traditional physicians steeped in its literature—about validating a competitive, free therapy with no undesirable side effects. Understandable.

Therefore, I would like to share my qualitative experiences that came about because of my recovery from a potentially terminal diagnosis. I would like to share what energy healing methods I favored, keeping in mind that the combinations of healing approaches I used, together and separately, all ultimately recharged my life-force energy.

I have certifications as a Reiki master, a hypnotherapist, and a Heart Touch hospice volunteer, in addition to my nursing degrees. I have also independently researched and participated in other energy healing practices without becoming formally certified. I especially like HeartMath, Energy Freedom Technique, and Quantum-Touch, but although I've experienced sessions and read about those practices, I am not qualified to hold forth with any great authority on them. I will leave further investigation up to the inquiring reader. There are a lot of different approaches to the same goal, all of them as valid as the students' intentions for learning.

Energy Freedom Technique, or EFT, is commonly known as tapping. It's a method for swiftly resolving emotional distress simply by tapping the fingertips on acupuncture energy meridian points. To the EFT aficionado, it can be practiced to improve all aspects of human behavior. I think it's worth further exploration, which is beyond the scope of this book. I noticed it shares similarities with shiatsu, Reiki, and yoga. I have to confess that I use my very limited tapping repertoire more as a first-aid technique than as an everyday preventative measure. I would benefit from using it more regularly, but I haven't made that leap yet.

HeartMath merits a lot of consideration. I attended a meeting in 2016 where the speaker was a HeartMath instructor. My notes say that HeartMath involves the energy reading of the human heart. Reportedly, when that frequency is in love/life mode, the reading corresponds to the background noise reading of the universe. It was said on September 11, 2001, the vibration of the collective hearts of humankind changed in response to the terrorist attack on New York City—as did the vibration of the universe, in a direct mirroring pattern. I didn't write in my notes by what means that measurement was done, but

I'm sure it can be ascertained. The theory was given that the heart, like the gut, has its own "brain." Well, I understand both the heart and gut release neurotransmitters, so I consider that a valid metaphor. Anyway, their premise is that an individual's heart rhythm can affect others and, by extrapolation, the world and the universe. That's getting into entanglement theory and way above the parameters of my mission here.

Hypnotherapy was my first course of study in mind over matter. Before I explored formal training in Reiki, I took an extended certification course in hypnotherapy. Hypnotherapy is a practice based on the energy of our minds. I find the innate ability to decide to voluntarily put oneself in an altered state of consciousness without any outside intervention to be an incredible gift. Even when there is someone else conducting a hypnosis session, keep in mind that the person is merely saying words and the subject is processing them and deciding how to react to them. The more you practice self-hypnosis—and all hypnosis is self-hypnosis, really—the quicker and deeper into relaxation you will go. You can put your "ego mind" on pause and contact your subconscious for all manner of information, all without pharmaceutical interference and its unwanted side effects. I think that self-hypnosis should be part of the required curriculum in school as a life skill, just like reading, writing, and arithmetic (especially now when computers can do all three of those for you).

Quantum-Touch is an energetic love-centered practice that evolved from polarity energy balancing as a system for healing as perceived and enhanced by Richard Gordon, who I think is a natural-born healer seeking to teach others how to unlock their natural healing abilities. Quantum-Touch is a powerful energy healing technique that works with life-force energy—a universal vibration of love and well-being. Also known as *chi* in Chinese and *prana* in Sanskrit, life-force energy is the flow of energy that sustains all living beings. Similar to Reiki, the energy exchange can involve physical touch or not and is holistic in scope, with unconditional love as its motivating intent.

There are a multitude of good books and internet offerings available about **Reiki**, which explain its history and philosophy and show the hand positions and symbols. This used to be considered secret, to keep knowledge and abilities available only to elitist groups. The rituals are probably useful for distracting our primitive brain/mind from blocking the energy. I'm going to go rogue here. It is stated in these texts that you must be attuned by someone. Baloney. Who attuned Dr. Usui, the founder? I was attuned three times by three different masters. One experience was extraordinary, as far as my feeling energy. The other two were unremarkable by my rather high standards. Do not let the "need to be attuned" prevent you from practicing on yourself what the books or videos teach. Especially lovely is Dr. Usui's original version of "The Reiki Ideals." If you want to go beyond self-care, then I recommend professional training. I consider Reiki to be a good foundational healing energy practice

Since Reiki is an area I have experience with, here's a little Reiki self-care practice called gassho meditation, which is used in Reiki to increase one's energy and promote a meditative frame of mind. The word "gassho" is a Japanese word that can be translated as meaning "two hands coming together." Gassho has elements of yoga and Zen and isn't as portable a breathing technique as some of the other breathing exercises in this book. Its purpose is to bring in healing energy through body position, breathing, and intention.

Affirmation Examples:

"I love all people and all people love me, and
I am continually bathed in the healing
energy of unconditional love."

"Universal good and healing is my only reality.
I am allowing life-force energy to restore and refresh my
entire being spiritually, mentally, and physically."

"My radiant health cannot be opposed, and I am
motivated to attain and maintain health and
balance in all aspects of my life."

Healing Exercise:

Sit down with your spine as straight as is comfortable, with closed eyes and hands placed together at heart level, similar to a prayer position. Focus your complete attention at the point where the two middle fingers meet. If it is uncomfortable to keep your hands in this position for several minutes (suggestions are anywhere from 5 to 30 minutes), keep them together and let them sink into your lap in a comfortable position and continue to meditate. You may experience your spine or hands becoming warm—don't let this bother you, just keep your focus on your two middle fingers. You can do this lying down, too, but there's always the invitation to sleep when in that position.

Inhale slowly through your nose, with your tongue pressed lightly against the top of your mouth just behind your front teeth, imagining life-force energy flowing through your crown chakra (the top of your head) along with air into your diaphragm. Hold your breath comfortably for a few seconds, imagining the energy spreading throughout your body. Now, let your jaw relax and rest your tongue on the bottom of your mouth as you exhale through your mouth.

Continue the breathing cycles slowly and easily until you feel you've received the benefit you want at this time. Close with a deep breath and a thank you, open your eyes, and be well.

It is recommended to perform gassho meditation daily, and it is purported that 15 minutes of gassho meditation is equivalent to a full-body Reiki self-treatment. Since I really like shortcuts, I highly recommend that. Fifteen minutes a day is a doable habit for an energetic tune-up.

As with all breathing exercises, be careful if you have any medical issues like asthma or high blood pressure. Follow the wisdom of your body and the counsel of your physician to determine if a technique is right for you or not.

Keep your suggestions positive. The subconscious is very literal and filters out negatives. It also is not confined by time parameters. Your subconscious is always awake, so be mindful of comments you make in everyday waking speech that it may take as suggestions.

Follow-Up Thoughts:

Again, there are tons of books, recordings, and qualified teachers to teach you self-hypnosis. Use whatever method suits you best, but I really do recommend acquiring the skill. It's very empowering to tap into your inborn ability to be the master of your own mind. What I would like to do here—since I don't have the space or inclination to go into a full-blown mini course on self-hypnosis—is to share some helpful hints related to the process.

They are mirroring a behavior you want to change in yourself, so use the interaction for self-reflection. You can't change them anyway, so use the opportunity for self-improvement. When you notice you are feeding your subconscious negativity, just turn it around. We're not perfect—we all do it. Personally, I apologize to myself, forgive myself, and then reframe the comment positively. It may sound like a silly game, but it works for me. One of my affirmations includes that I am immune to negativity from any source, including myself.

Making self-hypnosis suggestions for post-hypnotic behavior takes preparation. We don't naturally think and speak positively—it's an acquired technique. Usually, we know what we don't want, but we need to declare what we do want. It's just like writing affirmations, which are subconscious suggestions made while awake. Keep it personal, positive, and in the present tense.

I think I should mention here that you're not asleep in hypnosis. You are in a state of deep physical relaxation and heightened mental concentration. Because we are so literally suggestible in that state, I preface my suggestions with the disclaimer "If it is for my highest and best good, I am now…" just because I don't know every possible consequence of my consciously desired self-betterment.

Another interesting thing about hypnosis is that it can access your complete memory, because the subconscious never forgets. Additionally, we've all been spontaneously self-hypnotized zillions of times, slipping into a light or medium trance state while daydreaming, attending religious ceremonies, or concentrating on some activity like reading or watching media. A trance state is a natural phenomenon and nothing to be afraid of. It's just helpful to recognize being in a state of heightened suggestibility and realizing that you are always in charge of your acceptance of the messages.

The practice of touching people in the healing process is currently, during illnesses or pandemics, frowned upon. This may or may not be an unfortunate overreaction to the contagious nature of the virus. However, there is scientific validation for energy transference from one person to another without physical touch, so virtual hugs are worthwhile. Reiki and other energetic modalities do include the practice of distance healing. Of course, energetic distance healing has been going on for eons. It's called praying.

The energy of unconditional love is said to be the greatest healer of all. It is an experience that language is inadequate to describe. We can set the intention but its manifestation is mysterious, for as soon as we make an effort to feel it again it tends to elude us. Still the memory of it remains, and the desire to feel it again motivates us. Its power comes from loving for the sake of loving, without any expectation of reciprocity in any form. When we are able to access that energy, however briefly and through whatever technique, we prove to ourselves that it truly exists. And that's all that matters.

"For breath is life, so if you breathe well
you will live long on Earth."

—SANSKRIT PROVERB

CHAPTER FOUR
Breathing

Exploration of Healing Techniques
That Can Shift Your Energy

B REATHING IS ESSENTIAL TO PHYSICAL LIFE. We do it roughly 25,000 times a day. We are an oxygen-dependent species. What is magical is that before we're born, our bodies get oxygen from our mother's placental circulation; after the umbilical cord has been severed following birth, fully functional lungs, which have been bathed in fluid previously, switch over to using air to supply oxygen to our bodies. Amazing process.

Breathing techniques have a long history in spiritual practices in India and China, such as yoga and qigong. Hindu, Daoist, and Buddhist traditions regard control over breathing not only as essential for living, but also for spiritual growth. It is an idea that is also shared in some Islamic and Christian traditions. Today, we see the globalization of various viruses that attack our ability to breathe. No spiritual technique is available to keep control over our breathing.

Most of the modern breathwork therapies used today got their start during the consciousness-raising era of the 1960s and '70s, and they continue to evolve through different programs, scientific research, and studies. "Breathwork" is a general term used to describe any type of therapy that utilizes changes in the breathing pattern to improve mental, physical, and spiritual well-being.

There sure are a lot of suggestions out there on how to consciously change something like breathing that is automatic if we don't think about it. If we try to stop breathing voluntarily, our body's defense mechanism will kick in and make us breathe. If we stop breathing involuntarily, without heroic intervention, our bodies cease functioning completely.

Healthy babies breathe correctly. Watch a baby. They are obligate nose-breathers, and they breathe into their abdomen. How is it that we unconsciously alter that perfect pattern in response to environmental or psychological factors and then transform the very basic act of breathing into a bad habit?

Breath is life for our bodies. Everything comes after that. There are underappreciated health-care professionals called respiratory therapists whose job is to make sure patients are breathing properly. Inhaling brings in the new oxygen supply our cells require, and exhaling blows out the carbon dioxide that is a product of the chemical process of cellular respiration. This gas exchange takes place in the capillaries at the base of our lungs. Our noses are supplied with little hairs that filter out undesirable particles from the air we breathe, and our diaphragms push down and create a vacuum for air to fill the bottom of our lungs.

Many of us find ourselves, over the course of time, breathing shallowly through our mouths. The causes for this can range from the repetitive stress of daily life or poor posture to chronic disease states. This "chest breathing" is a habit that can be changed by relearning how to breathe into the diaphragm through our noses. Relaxed "belly breathing" encourages the best exchange of oxygen and carbon dioxide and can slow the heartbeat and lower blood pressure.

Okay, so much for our mini clinical review.

It doesn't matter which is your favorite, or if you feel you are already breathing properly. Paying attention to thoughtful breathing, especially under challenging conditions, can give you a boost, and changing your breathing can change your mood. Different breathing practices come from a variety of sources and are sometimes gathered together as "breathwork techniques." The practice of yoga is particularly rich with breathing techniques, and I'm pretty sure most of breathwork evolved from yoga breathing techniques made popular after India's remarkable impact on Western culture, beginning in the 18th century.

This section contains a few key breathing exercises for you to enjoy and hopefully practice. These are just a sampling of breathing techniques that I used to restore my body to wellness and which I continue to practice daily, and they are not a comprehensive collection of breathwork techniques. Their origins run the gamut from basic respiratory therapy to the yogic practice of breath regulation called pranayama.

Deep Abdominal Breathing—This is just what it sounds like. You breathe deeply into your abdomen, allowing both your chest and belly to expand as far as you can manage. Getting full expansion of your lungs is a good thing, and very helpful should you ever need a chest X-ray. When you exhale fully, your body relaxes. Many of the other techniques assume you are breathing deeply into your abdomen, so it's good to practice.

Box Breathing—Named for the 4-4-4-4 count that could be visualized as a box or square, this is also called Four-Square Breathing. You breathe in, hold, exhale, and rest, each to the same count of 4. Very easy to learn and do, and good for calming down quickly after a stressful experience. If you only want to practice one breathing technique, this is the one. It is taught to the military, and repeated, regular practice may positively change how the body reacts to stress.

Alternate Nostril Breathing—This is a yoga technique to encourage mind/body balance. It helps to balance the right and left hemispheres of the brain. It takes a bit of practice to get all the moving parts coordinated, but I find it useful for grounding prior to meditation.

4-7-8 Breathing—This is the count for the inhalation, hold, and exhalation. Also called the Relaxing Breath in yoga practice, it's used for deep relaxation, so it's not recommended during stressful activities that require focus and attention, like driving or operating heavy equipment. This is best reserved for going to sleep. I have found it very effective for going back to sleep after something wakes me up.

Lamaze Breathing—I reference this method because it was really the gateway practice to conscious breathing for me, and many people are familiar with it. It also appears to be yoga-inspired. Dr. Fernand Lamaze taught the Lamaze method in his clinic in Paris, and Americans who gave birth there brought it back to America in the 1960s. The Lamaze method did originally have specific breathing patterns and guidelines, but now it's just controlled, slow, deep breathing that feels right to you. There is no "right" way and no rules related to how many breaths per minute or whether to breathe through the nose or mouth or make sounds. You may focus on something to maintain the rhythm of your breathing, if you wish. The main thing is that your breathing is conscious, not automatic. Controlled, conscious, slow, deep breathing increases oxygenation, relaxation, and mindfulness. Lamaze breathing seems to have evolved into a form of laissez-faire yoga breathing.

Affirmation Examples:

"I am keeping myself in the now.
Just breathing and healing."

"I am breathing in my own empowering, healing light."

"As I breathe in my calmness, I breathe out
all my stress."

Healing Exercise:

Let's start with a health-care-oriented basic exercise for **diaphragmatic (belly) breathing**. This is a variation of the breathing used in the centering process.

Lie on your back on your bed or other comfortable flat surface. Bend your knees. Put a pillow under your knees and one under your head for comfort.

Place one hand on your belly just under your rib cage and the other on your upper chest.

Breathe deeply and slowly through your nose into your abdomen. The hand on your belly should rise and the hand on your chest should not.

Contract your abdominal muscles to expel the air and exhale through pursed lips. ("Pursed lips" tutorial: Pucker your lips like you were going to whistle. Don't force the air out. Breathe out gently and deliberately, breathing out longer than it took you to breathe in. Counting helps.) The hand on your belly should go down.

You can also practice this sitting straight in a chair, knees bent, feet on the floor if comfortable, with your shoulders and neck relaxed.

After you've gotten the technique down, this can be done anytime, anywhere, in any position, without needing to use your hands to verify you're breathing into your belly.

My suggestion is to do this exercise for 5 to 10 minutes, 4 or 5 times daily if possible. If that seems like a lot, do the best you can.

Now that you have refreshed yourself with belly breathing, which is pretty much the foundation of other breathing techniques, we can touch on some exercises for specific benefits.

Sit in a safe, comfortable position—you know the drill. Tilt your chin up slightly to improve airflow, then breathe in deeply through your nose and exhale for twice as long as you inhaled. This is a cycle. A set of 4 repetitions of the cycle once or twice a day is good for circulation.

For good digestion, before dinner take 5 minutes to practice breathing deeply into your belly, making your abdomen rise fully, and then exhale slowly as long as you can, tightening your abdominal muscles to push out the air.

Okay, how about a breathing technique that is useful to alleviate stress and anxiety?

This technique is alternate nostril breathing (called nadi shodhana in Sanskrit, for inquiring minds who want to know). It's uncomfortable for me to position my hands and fingers in the correct yoga positions, so I freestyle and I've omitted those instructions. Feel free to look them up.

Use the thumb and fourth finger of your dominant hand to gently close off one nostril at a time while you are exhaling and inhaling out of the other.

You are going to inhale and exhale only through the nose. At first, this may feel a little odd and restrictive. Just relax and get into a comfortable rhythm. You don't have to take really deep breaths. Breathe at your normal rate, slow and easy, making sure your shoulders are staying relaxed. Try practicing doing this for a minute or two. Once you have it down, you have another tool for calm you can use anytime. If it makes you lightheaded, release both nostrils and breathe normally. If you're congested, you may need tissues nearby.

First, gently block your right nostril and inhale through your left nostril into your belly. Hold your breath while you unblock the right nostril and block the left.

Exhale through your right nostril and then inhale through it. Hold the breath while you unblock the left nostril and block the right. Exhale through the left, inhale through the left.

Repeat this pattern where you exhale then inhale on the same side, hold briefly, unblock the exhale side, and block the inhale side in alternate order.

When I first started using this technique, it was a bit bizarre, like using an air neti pot, but it really does bring your attention to your breath and relaxes you. Maybe because you have to concentrate and be coordinated with your breath and your thumb and fourth finger, like you're playing a musical instrument. I don't know if I need to add that I practice this exercise discreetly. It's not really appropriate for performance art.

Alrighty then, let's move on. How about trying the 4-7-8 breathing technique that is reported to help one get to sleep? There's a theory that the conscious mind can only handle two tasks simultaneously, so if you can otherwise occupy it, the monkey mind will surrender to sleep. It is a variation on counting sheep, but instead you're counting breaths.

As an aside, if you're having trouble getting to sleep and staying asleep, additional new (boring) bedtime habits may help. All are optional. Feel free to mix and match or ignore altogether. Go to bed (early enough to get at least 7 hours of sleep) and wake up around the same time 7 days a week, 52 weeks a year. In other words, all the time, even weekends, holidays, and vacations. Keep your bedroom cool and dark. Avoid electronics that emit a blue light in the evening. Don't let your pet sleep with you. Don't eat within two hours of retiring for the night, unless it's a light, healthy snack. Avoid alcohol before bedtime and limit fluid intake. It should take from 10 to 20 minutes to fall asleep, and your heart rate should be below 60. Doing the following Relaxing Breath exercise can help. Yes, it's derived from yoga, which is why it is referred to as the 4-7-8 breathing technique.

To first get the hang of the technique, sit with your back straight. Of course, if you want to get to sleep at night, you'd do it in bed, but we're just practicing here. Place the tip of your tongue against the roof of your mouth just behind your front teeth and keep it there throughout the exercise. You will be exhaling around your tongue. Pursing your lips slightly during the exhale can help keep your tongue in the proper position. To begin, with your tongue in place, part your lips and exhale completely through your mouth making a "whoosh" sound. Then close your lips and inhale quietly through your nose to the count of 4 in your head. Hold your breath for a mental count of 7. Exhale through your mouth to a count of 8, making the "whoosh" sound.

This is one breath cycle. Repeat for 3 more breath cycles, for a total of 4. Do it at least twice a day. You can do it more frequently, but only do 4 breath cycles at a time and remember it's to help you go to sleep. Practice, practice, practice. You can work your way up to 8 breath cycles after a month or so, but no more than that in one sitting. Note to self: This technique is very good for sleep, and so it should not be practiced in a setting where you're not safe to fully relax and/or need to be completely alert immediately after practicing. As in, this is not the practice to use to relax while driving in traffic.

With all breathing exercises, be careful if you have any medical issues like asthma or high blood pressure. Follow the wisdom of your body and the counsel of your physician to determine if a technique is right or not for you.

You may be wondering about the tongue placement thing. I was, so I looked it up. It has to do with stimulating your vagus nerve, which originates in your brain stem and extends all the way down to the tongue, vocal chords, heart, lungs, digestive system, and other internal organs. It is the most important component of your parasympathetic nervous system: the one that calms you down. The vagal response reduces stress. Deep, complete belly breathing is an agreed upon best practice for stimulating your vagus nerve. The tongue and the soft and hard palate (roof of your mouth) are other areas of stimulation, hence positioning your tongue against your hard palate during breathing exercises. This also connects to proper tongue posture (who knew there was such a thing?), which is to have your tongue pressed against the roof of your mouth behind your teeth and not resting on the bottom of your mouth. The front tip of your tongue should be about a half inch from your front teeth. I just learned about this and plan to practice when I notice my lazy tongue lounging on the bottom of my mouth, because I have developed a swallowing problem that may be related to poor tongue posture. Chin up!

Lastly, there's the tried-and-true box breathing technique, easy peasy and can be practiced discreetly. Assume the position: Sit up straight, feet flat on floor, hands in your lap with palms facing up. Slowly exhale, emptying your lungs completely. Inhale slowly through your nose for the count of 4, filling your lungs with air as with belly breathing. Pause and hold your breath for the same count of 4. Exhale through your mouth for an equal count of 4, and then again pause and hold your breath for a count of 4 before repeating the cycle. This exercise is good to practice 5 minutes a day just to have that behavior memory to call upon when stressful events pop up out of nowhere and cause anxiety. You can say no to panic and yes to peace. Just breathe.

Follow-Up Thoughts:

Here's a catchy saying from nursing, where low moods can show up with regularity and dark humor with a double meaning is the norm: "Whenever I feel blue, I start breathing again." Knowing you have an easy personal tool available like controlling your breathing, which can positively impact your outlook on life immediately, is immensely powerful. Not surprisingly, mindful breathing is also included in several psychological, spiritual, and religious practices. Very holistic.

"Forgive yourself for not knowing
then what you know now."

—MAYA ANGELOU

CHAPTER FIVE

Forgiveness and Gratitude

Using Divine Unconditional Love to Help
Restore Your Health and Freedom

ORGIVENESS REDIRECTS OUR ATTENTION from the past and allows us to be fully present in the now. Maya Angelou (1928–2014) was an American poet, performer, and world-famous author. She had an amazing variety of experiences in the course of her long life, some of which were decidedly unpleasant.

> "Let gratitude be the pillow upon which you
> kneel to say your nightly prayer."
> —Maya Angelou

She wrote numerous autobiographies detailing her education on schoolhouse Earth, and I admire her shared wisdom very much. The quotes from Maya Angelou remind me of the two faces on the tragedy and comedy masks that are the symbol for theater, which represent opposing sides of the human emotional range. They are the bookends for our library of life lessons. Love is the capstone of the learning pyramid, and forgiveness and gratitude are the two supporting blocks underneath.

Every human interaction is an experience. Nothing more, nothing less. How we choose to interpret the outcome of those experiences is up to us. We are imperfect human beings doing the best we can, and sometimes our personal best offends someone. We are not responsible for their feelings. We can certainly acknowledge those feelings exist. But we don't own anyone else's feelings. We need to mind our own business and conduct ourselves with our best version of personal morality and ethics.

If you accept that everything in the Universe is a gift freely given by the Source of All Creation, then gratitude should be fairly automatic. Something started the ball rolling, and it would be bad form not to say "Thank you." There is an opinion attributed to German philosopher and mystic Meister Eckhart that if the only prayer you ever say is "Thank you," that's enough. A new mantra going around currently is "Thank you for the gift of that experience." Because even when good days make you happy, not so good days give you experience, and it's all a gift.

Gratitude doesn't just apply to divine interventions. Marcus Tullius Cicero said, "Gratitude is not only the greatest of virtues, but the parent of all others." Fellow humans can be generous with their time, talent, and money, so gratitude can also be expressed as appreciation for their contributions to your life. We are taught from our earliest years to say "Thank you" when receiving a gift and, as we get older, to make a habit of expressing gratitude to others, because silent gratitude doesn't acknowledge the other person's loving kindness out loud, either in word or deed. They can reply, "Oh, it was nothing," which may indicate they were giving unconditionally, but it doesn't pertain to their reciprocal gratitude for the act of being valued. The energy of gratitude continues to radiate exponentially, improving the world one "Thank you" at a time.

Gratitude is as simple as forgiveness is complex.

True forgiveness is an interesting concept, like sacred selfishness. Forgiveness has two identities—one from the purely material point of view and one from the Big Picture view of life on Earth.

In the realm of materiality, humans seem to have this deep-seated need to forgive and be forgiven by each other and their community in order to not be excluded. Exclusion can take many forms, from the "silent treatment" to current social media "cancel culture." This aversion to missing out is understandable. Historically, to be excluded was potentially a death sentence. Fear of abandonment follows us around, making us believe we're not worthy of being included in the group, be it family, friend groups, school, workplace, clubs, associations, etc. Major organized religions promise redemption through Divine forgiveness, and that tenet resonates with millions of adherents. The belief is that the separation is of the individual from the Divine, which was evidently voluntary and a bad move but will be remedied by atonement. Eventually.

As regards the Big Picture or metaphysical life philosophy, the Source is not a judge—whatever It is, It is not anthropomorphic (having human characteristics), and judgment is a result of human emotions playing with reason and logic.

Human-centered forgiveness ultimately deals with a victim mentality, although there are many experts who would argue that type of forgiveness frees you from victimhood. From personal experience, I can tell you there are many, many books, speakers, and seminars that all revolve around reinforcing letting go of the resentment one has developed because of another's behavior. And they can be helpful in sorting out feelings and emotions that no longer serve us. As with unanticipated change, we have no control over the actions of others. Our control, such as it is, is limited to our judgment of the behavior of others and our reaction to it.

Hawaiian culture has a beautiful practice for reconciliation with the Divine within us all, called the Ho'oponopono: "I'm sorry. Please forgive me. Thank you. I love you." The Ho'oponopono also offers thanks for whatever experience occurred. That is a lovely prayer, as long as it doesn't put the power of forgiveness outside oneself, where it doesn't really belong. No one else can forgive us. That is how the popular conception of forgiveness endorses the victim archetype, which is the human race's bad habit of attacking and defending against one another.

To forgive is divine. It comes from the divine spark within each of us and is concerned with forgiving ourselves. Forgiveness is a spiritual quality because it overrides our human response to avenge a perceived wrong. Forgiveness assumes a moral circumspection that extends beyond the animal instinct to fight for property, food, and safety. We have no dominion over others that gives us the power or the right to bestow forgiveness. Forgiveness implies that we know another's heart, motivations, and life lessons and that we have the wherewithal to absolve them from their transgressions. Can't do that. Theirs is not our story to critique or edit.

Let's look at the situation objectively. You have decided that someone has angered, hurt, disappointed, or otherwise irritated you. Or you assume that you have (on purpose or inadvertently) angered, hurt, or disappointed someone, as though you have the power to make others your emotional marionette. What's wrong with this picture?

I recall, with a lot of discomfort, having a conversation with my mother near the end of her life. She confided in me she had had an emotional, healing breakthrough and that she had finally forgiven herself. My mother had been a serial, relapsing alcoholic, who also commented without irony that she was always the oldest person in her AA group. In my callous, middle-aged mind, I thought then that it would have been nicer at this stage of our relationship for her to apologize to me and ask my forgiveness for all the shit she'd put me through for my entire life. That wasn't happening. Now, as I approach the age she was when she told me that, I understand more clearly that she was offering me one last life lesson before she exited stage left.

Observe your less-than-stellar behavior with the understanding, compassion, and grace that you would nonjudgmentally use in observing—but not condoning—the bad behavior of others. If we're informed that we've been the perpetrators of an insult, the courtesy of a sincere apology makes forgiveness of judgment easier for the other and for us. How's that for a double dose of potentially bitter medicine? It is the sweetness of mercy that allows the medicine to go down.

This is not to say that the exercises for forgiveness related to human-centered forgiveness are not helpful. They are short-term or intermediate fixes. If you have been the target of willful abuse, your first thoughts may not be to thank your abuser for the gift of that experience. It's not possible for most of humankind to be spiritual during or immediately following physical or psychological harm. Those people are called saints. We can't deny that evil experiences happen. Evil is the misuse of our power. Our power, or life energy, is inherently good. So, evil is not an independent thing, it results from an unwise choice. Experiences are energy in motion, and they have consequences.

This theory shows that forgiveness doesn't condone the bad behavior of others, but if you carry anger and resentment about it, that reaction will harm you further. Human forgiveness involves severing any negative connections that bind you to the perpetrator of the perceived insult, thus freeing yourself. It's best not to judge the experience as good or bad—it was just an experience that can generate positive or negative feelings or can be neutralized completely. You can use your free will to choose your reaction. We can distill our lives into a collection of experiences by which we learn how better to love ourselves and others.

There is a saying that what bothers us about others is what bothers us most about ourselves. Someone's upsetting behavior will trigger memories of similar circumstances in our past, because memory is annoying that way. If a situation has made us uncomfortable, it is a signal that something in our life is out of whack. We are being given an opportunity to notice something that needs healing attention. Occasionally, the message has to be loud and insistent because we've been shining it on. In my case, it took a potentially life-threatening illness to get my full attention.

Here's a silly story about a man who was always snapping his fingers. A friend asked him why he did that. He replied that it kept the elephants away. His friend said that there weren't any elephants anywhere near them. The man smiled and said, "See, it's working." My takeaway from that is that it's better to continually practice forgiveness than to have to struggle to restart the habit when a resentment the size of an elephant is sitting on your chest.

What does continual forgiveness improvement look like? Simply put, it is choosing love over judgment. We can conduct our lives with integrity and uphold our higher principles without having to prove we are "right" and someone else is "wrong." We can reinforce the belief that we are enough. We can allow ourselves at any time during our life to reassess and choose a different path. There is always an alternative. We can step back and observe situations, acknowledging that underneath all the apparent circumstances, love exists there. We can be okay with not knowing everything and realize that people will violate societal agreements on behavior for their own reasons. However, safeguards do need to be in place and enforced by the government for the common good, because we have the right to expect adherence to agreed-upon behavioral boundaries. If we act from the motivation of what is for the highest good, the energy of that love will radiate like the ripples in a pond when a stone is dropped in it.

Let forgiveness go on autopilot. Don't try to forgive; just affirm it and let its energy do its thing without your interference. This is the real basis of forgive and forget.

We don't forget to pretend some injury did not happen. We forget to keep ourselves from constantly reliving the past and keeping negative emotions connected to the past in the present. Populations and countries have pasts that are filled with unresolved conflicts brought forward into the present because new generations are taught that they are victims and should be resentful about them. This type of tradition needs to stop. There is a great need for individuals and societies to heal the past so they can move forward. We need to do a fearless moral inventory and make amends as long as it would not cause injury. In recognizing that we've taken a detour, we can always make a course correction and get back on track. Make peace with the past so it doesn't interfere with the future, and we can joyously live in the now.

Here's the thing: All forgiveness is self-forgiveness. This seems counterintuitive in our victim-oriented culture. The actions of others do not determine our destiny. Those actions may reroute our path, but they don't define our destiny. We do not need the empathy of others to validate our self-imposed suffering, no matter how comfortingly familiar it feels. Don't be a prisoner of your past in a dungeon of your own making. Let go of the survival patterns you either were taught or made up that no longer serve you. Change your assumption that what happened was personal. Forgive yourself for needing a past experience in order to have compassionate insight now. Others are going to do what they're going to do and you can't stop the train wreck, even if you see it coming and know it will affect you. Choose serenity, courage, and wisdom. We are all interconnected, so we don't have to take it personally. Ultimately, forgiveness is being at peace with being imperfect.

Affirmation Examples:

"I am endlessly forgiving and free."

"I show gratitude for my family, my friends, and my abundant health."

"I am overflowing with gratitude as I let go and demonstrate forgiveness."

Healing Exercise:

You can formulate your own affirmation or modify one you've discovered. The Ho'oponopono can be very powerful when addressed to yourself. There is also an ancient Indigenous Central American blessing that says, in part, "Learning through love, I bless my way of expressing, even though someone may not understand me."

Follow-Up Thoughts:

The theory of cause and effect claims that for every effect (results or outcome) there was a cause that contributed to that effect—and, I would like to add, even when we don't know what the cause was, why it happened, or what good can come of it. When expressing gratitude, you can always say, "Thank you for the gift of that experience." Time may or may not put it into perspective, but gratitude is better than resentment. No one ever got sick because they were thankful.

"A good laugh and a long sleep are the
two best cures for anything."

—IRISH PROVERB

CHAPTER SIX

Eating, Laughing, Relaxing

Transforming Everyday Behaviors into
Loving and Healing Actions

L ET'S CIRCLE BACK TO THE PREMISE of this healing work, which is to engage in radical loving self-care to restore you back to your natural and empowered self. We've touched on a holistic approach, sacred selfishness, energy work, breathing, gratitude, and forgiveness.

A conventional part of self-care for health involves nutrition, movement, touching, and sleep, so a brief shout-out to those topics is in order. The world is flooded with good and not-so-good advice on those subjects. Back in the day, when I was an RN Certified Diabetes Educator, my emphasis was on creating lifestyle plans my clients would actually stick to because they were doable and borderline enjoyable. An important note: I coached people who had been diagnosed with type 2 diabetes. Insulin-dependent type 1 diabetes is a whole different care plan. They have similarities, but as far as I'm concerned, in my opinion, type 1 is an autoimmune disorder and type 2 is a digestive repetitive-stress disorder.

A brief personal disclaimer before I launch into Nancy Nurse on nutrition. For as long as I can remember, I have had a love-hate relationship with food. I couldn't be bothered with food when I was a child. My mother said on many occasions that if I didn't like peanut butter and jelly sandwiches with chocolate milk, I would not have survived. I was beyond a picky eater. I wasn't interested in eating at all, because it would interrupt my preferred activities. However, when I did eat, I could out-eat my older brothers and not gain an ounce. After puberty, my appetite picked up to the point that I became overweight after I stopped participating in sports. So, from about age 16 on, it seems like I've been dieting, one way or another. Yes, I know the word "diet" contains the word "die." I also know if you program your subconscious to lose weight, it will seek to find it again. Better verbiage is following a lifelong healthy eating plan and permanently getting rid of unnecessary excess fat so that we can be healthy, fit, and trim.

I must admit, when I was unwell with my recent digestive issues, I actually became afraid of food. A fear-based existence is just a crappy way to live. I got out of it, and so can you. That's kind of the purpose of this book.

Anyway, I didn't know how my body would react to foods that had previously been tasty, fun, and healthy. By that point in my life, eating had become my primary pleasure, and then food couldn't be trusted not to compromise my social acceptability, if you catch my meaning. The inability to control bodily functions in public is definitely frowned upon. If I had had the exhaustive surgery that was being recommended, I would have faced an even worse digestive scenario, because it would have permanently removed important parts with no chance of the system ever repairing itself. So, if eating makes you anxious, I totally understand. Food is necessary, so we need to make it our friend, not our foe. It's a thoughtful practice to be grateful for our food and acknowledge how lucky we are to be in an abundant position to choose healthy food items and portion sizes.

A good start is to differentiate between real food that provides nutrition and edible substances that are nonnutritious or of low nutritional value except for being "enriched" after processing. While there are no inherently evil foods, I do differentiate between natural nutritious food and edible items that provide limited or no nutrition and don't seem to poison you immediately.

The Standard American Diet (SAD) has been heavily influenced by advertising from processed food manufacturers who are in the business to make a profit, not to make us healthy. Here's an easy rule of thumb: Eat real food, only cooked as necessary for your digestive system to process.

Organic, if possible; non-GMO for sure. Don't challenge me on genetically modified organisms being okay. GMO is not hybridizing and/or doing selective breeding within the same plant or animal. It is splicing genes from one species and inserting them into the nucleus of another so that the result will express desired marketable characteristics. It is Frankenstein food, and we do not yet have long-term data showing how eating products of genetic manipulation will affect our bodies—plant and animal genes are in play together there.

I understand many people can't afford to buy only organic food, but we don't need another food experiment to increase stockholder profits performed on our bodies. We're still not completely sure how pesticides and food additives are impacting the overall health of humanity, but it doesn't look wonderful. There are still starving people all over the world, so increased productivity doesn't rationalize it. Enough said.

Refrain from putting a lot of fat, salt, and sugar where they weren't originally. Adding fat, salt, and sugar in a precise ratio is a strategy that purveyors of fast food and junk food excel at because it triggers addictive consumption of their products. Eating mostly plants is a good idea as long as you can get sufficient vitamin B_{12} from some clean source. Personally, I'm OK with organic free-range eggs and a supplement that also contains intrinsic factors and folic acid recommended to me by my gastroenterologist, who happens to be vegan. I also occasionally eat wild-caught fish and organic dairy products like yogurt and cheese. But that's just me.

I guess I could be labeled a flexitarian, if you're into labels. There's no one-size-fits-all, as far as an eating plan goes. Chew your carbohydrates and combine them with fiber. There are a lot of good sources you can use in order to create an eating plan that suits you. Rule of thumb in choosing dietary advice: Follow the money. I know it's a pain but check out who paid for the research that's being used as the basis for a specific eating plan and who makes a profit from people following it. Don't let perfect get in the way of good, but do be responsibly informed and act according to the best of your ability.

As for movement, 30 minutes a day of directed activity is probably a minimum to keep your muscles hungry for the circulating sugar in your blood. Do whatever you enjoy. Walk, dance, swim, do chair yoga, use gym equipment— just do a little every day. You don't have to do it all at once to get the benefit—you can walk 10 minutes three times a day—as long as the cumulative time spent is enough to use up some glucose in your muscles so that they'll take some circulating glucose out of your blood. Our bodies are designed to be physical and move, so make it a daily habit to exercise. Oh, and get some sunshine every day with appropriate sunscreen, or ask your doctor about taking a vitamin D3 supplement.

As a result of the COVD-19 pandemic, I've had to revise what I wrote in my original lesson plan about the importance of human touch. Touch is an especially important human sense, and the contagious aspect of the virus has seriously impacted it. Touch is the strongest nonverbal communication one can give another. Through touch, we are also sharing subtle energy because touch by its nature is reciprocal. Touch is essential for newborns, who will die if they are not touched. There have been studies on the health benefits of hugging. I'm a big fan of hugging to share the love, so the restraints caused by this pandemic are really challenging. Incorporate a plan to hug the people in your household every day. If you live alone and are in isolation, you can hug yourself; just fold your arms around your body in any way that feels comfortable and hug yourself for as long as you want. It's okay to rock back and forth when you do this. If you want a modified self-hug, stroke your arms from shoulder to hand, alternating sides. I give myself Reiki every day. Self-comfort is an expression of the compassion and loving kindness that is a cornerstone of radical loving self-care. When the COVID-19 situation was satisfactorily resolved, the first thing I did was to hug my family and friends with abandon.

As for sleep, I offered some tools in the breathing chapter. Insomnia is a problem for many people normally, and the stress of the pandemic can make it more pronounced. Fortunately for me, unless my body is severely out of balance,

I have always slept well. The purpose of this book is to help you bring your body back into balance, so sleep should be an appreciated side effect of the other health practices. To sleep like a baby is an appropriate goal. I don't consciously remember being a baby, but in observing them, it seems that once their physical needs are met—they're clean; fed; in comfortable, safe surroundings; and have been cuddled—they surrender to sleep rather easily. Adults are a little more complicated because we think too much. I'm certainly not an expert in this area, but personally, I find the 4-7-8 breathing pattern, the count for the inhalation, hold, and exhalation exercise I share in Chapter 4, calms me down enough to fall asleep.

I thought I had incorporated the holistic, complementary self-care practices I taught my clients into my daily life, but when I got sick, I reviewed them to discover where I had slacked off. It's always good to make sure one hasn't remembered something incorrectly, since it's human nature to modify and reinterpret instructions. I suggest you use some method to stay on course for your own health and wellness journey.

Consider making a checklist. I've found it's too easy to "forget" to do things that I know are in my own best interests because they're annoying for some reason. There's a place in our lizard brain that feels threatened by change, of course, but we have the tools to override any faulty programming. It's so weird, because the pandemic public health instructions are like an order to take care of yourself and others, yet people are rebelling against them and getting sick and dying because they don't want someone to order them around, even if it's for their own good. Freedom can be a contradictory concept.

Way back in 1975, the bestselling book *The Relaxation Response* by Herbert Benson, MD, was published and took the stressed-out working world by storm. The foreword states that this book is the result of combining recent science with older Eastern and Western writings to demonstrate that people naturally know how to relax. But just in case you've forgotten how, here's a few hundred pages of research and opinion to support the validity of practicing four elements for 10 to 20 minutes once or twice daily. The author recommends readers practice this relaxation technique, which he described as a person's inborn nature, only with the approval and supervision of their physician. Wow. Reading that disclaimer stressed me out.

My opinion is that the book was a well-intentioned, evidence-based introduction to intentionally integrating basic meditation into our health-care culture. Back then, we were trying to figure out how to deal with the shocking aftereffects of the 1960s—Nixon's presidency, the Vietnam War, civil rights, gay rights, women's rights, environmental issues, recreational drug use, etc. There was a lot to worry about, and it seemed to be negatively affecting our health. Not much has changed except the names in the past half century.

Now, this wasn't an entirely new idea. Hans Selye, MD, brought the word "stress" into medical terminology through his copious published research and his best-known book, *The Stress of Life*, published in 1956. In 1975, he was busy founding the International Institute of Stress and creating the Hans Selye Foundation.

Although the two doctors seem to have parallel paths, there is a fork in the road. Dr. Selye was concerned with the physical responses to acute stress caused by universal patient reactions to a diagnosed illness. He was branching out from prior health theories that the body is always trying to get back to systemic balance, or homeostasis. Dr. Benson was addressing the fight-or-flight response to perceived threats that doesn't resolve immediately after the threat passes. It is an unfortunate side effect of imagination. Imagination sometimes needs to be quieted if it is not serving us constructively. To to do this, we need to calm our mind.

Meditation is a way to alter our consciousness away from an overload of worrisome self-storytelling and toward quiet relaxation. A gentle reminder: Theoretically, the brain/mind can only handle two things at once. Thus, if one is doing mindful breathing and chanting a mantra, there's no room for pesky thoughts to rev up our sympathetic nervous system and let loose the adrenaline. When such thoughts intrude, we merely acknowledge them, dismiss them, and go back to what we were doing to support our parasympathetic nervous system, which is pro-relaxation. Sounds simple, but it's not so easy. We have to establish a new overriding habit pattern, which we'll go over in a different chapter.

Here's a little tale to explain the fight-or-flight reaction. A herd of antelope are grazing on the savannah. A pride of lions approaches on the hunt. The antelope evaluate the situation and either successfully flee, or they fight if caught and then flee or die. If the lions are successful in their hunt, the survivors relax and go back to grazing, because the real, immediate threat to life is over for now. The lions are full and have gone to sleep. The antelope doesn't stop eating normally, wandering around constantly worrying about the next inevitable lion hunt in a state of never-ending hypervigilance.

The moral of the story is that in our current technological society, lions will not stalk you, kill you, and eat you, but your primitive brain/mind doesn't know that unless you proactively instruct it otherwise. In our technological, industrialized culture, the part of the lions can be played by numerous actors: bosses, careless drivers, mean people— anyone or any circumstance that causes us anxiety. The trick is to relax after perceived close encounters by practicing techniques that bring our bodies back to baseline. What separates us from the animals is imagination.

We need so-called positive stress to survive. Otherwise, we would be immobile and starve to death. Stressors motivate us to take action, but being chronically overly sensitive to stressors leads to worry. Worrying is useless and can lead to anxiety, which can become debilitating. Things are going to happen the way they're going to happen, whether you worry about them or not. No amount of anxiety will change the outcome. Not that you shouldn't strategize for probable outcomes, accepting the fact that you can't prepare for everything. Worry is continually disturbing your peace of mind by fretting over things outside of your sphere of influence. It is a key healing exercise to change the story of your future by adapting to new information. If you are unable to change the circumstances of your life, you can change the way you think about them. There are too many variables to be an infallible fortune teller, but you do have the power to change your mind.

Allow me to address the worthlessness of worry from personal experience. My mother—may she rest in peace—told me I was born a worrier. I, on the other hand, think I was born a caregiver. My eldest daughter would tell her friends that she didn't need to worry about anything, because I would worry for her. I was the family's designated worrier. A side effect was that I was a pretty good planner, which is a euphemism for being a control freak.

Suffice it to say, what was going to happen was going to happen, whether I worried about it or not. My loved ones would occasionally get sick, be injured, and have their dreams shattered and their hearts broken. I could not protect myself from the slings and arrows of outrageous fortune, much less protect them, but that didn't keep me from being a helicopter mom of epic proportions. Thankfully, by their own choices, my children are loving, kind, compassionate human beings with well-developed senses of humor who survived my penchant for putting an "s" in front of mother for a good portion of their young lives because I was worried for them.

I cannot imagine how much more extreme my behavior might have been had I not learned self-hypnosis. Back in the day, my so-called relaxant of choice was alcohol. It wasn't until I realized it was affecting others beyond me that I decided to change. Alcohol is not a relaxant; it is a central nervous system depressant. It is a toxic solvent. I finally heeded the call to abstinence when I became pregnant, knowing that it would find its way not just into my nervous system, but my unborn child's system as well. That was my slap-in-the-face moment. In a prenatal Lamaze course, I discovered breathing and relaxation techniques that just aced the frantic daily affirmations and prayers in the drug-less bliss department.

I need to clarify that I was alcohol-free while pregnant and nursing. I could extend that courtesy for my children, but to be alcohol-free for just my own benefit would come a few years later. I started researching and reading books about the process, including the aforementioned *The Relaxation Response*, which had been recently published. I also studied Jess Stearn's *The Power of Alpha-Thinking*, published in 1976. Alpha-thinking is a kind of benevolent mix of self-hypnosis heavy in visualization and telepathy based on brain wave frequency. All I'm going to say about telepathy here is that if it was good enough for the KGB and the CIA, it's good enough for me. Six years went by before I could enroll in professional courses to become certified as a hypnotherapist. I birthed all three of my children without drugs and even had a root canal without the benefit of drugs, just using self-hypnosis.

Here's the deal: The pain in childbirth is mainly muscular contractions, and you can use relaxation techniques to not make it worse. However, a root canal involves a nerve that goes directly to your brain, so it's not merely a matter of muscle relaxation. To get something like that done under self-hypnosis requires you to put yourself in an altered state of consciousness that's just this side of an out-of-body experience. Maybe it would have been easier if the dentist who claimed to be trained in hypnosis supported me, but he seemed to lose his concentration in that area during the procedure. I made it through, but I do not recommend it. Sometimes the best course is to take the medicine. Just because you can do something doesn't mean you have to.

Anyway, it was an easy segue from self-hypnosis to meditation. They both involve relaxing the body. There are active behavior change suggestions involved in hypnosis for your subconscious to work on during your waking hours. Meditation is far more passive. You just sit, relax, and breathe. Thinking is not only not required, but it is clearly discouraged.

One thing that the study of hypnosis reveals is the realization that we are being bombarded constantly with suggestions that are timed to be applied during times of natural relaxation, when we are susceptible to subconscious input. Television advertisements are the most obvious, although the news media is becoming revenue-based propaganda, a sales pitch to buy one side's opinion rather than a free exchange of ideas or merely the reporting of observable and verifiable facts. Don't get me started on how politics is becoming a spectator sport, with rabid fans totally disconnected from the human consequences of their actions because they have accepted post-hypnotic suggestions. We are not only what we eat, but also what we allow our minds and emotions to feed on.

Here's a quick primer on the universal sales technique that speaks to your subconscious mind. Establish rapport with the customer by using a trust technique. Nudge your ego out of the way and be nonjudgmental (this is a hallmark of unconditional love). Actively listen. Make them feel valued, make sense in your presentation, and be thoughtful. Once rapport is established, determine what they're afraid of and tell them you're the only one who can save them.

Unfortunately, fear is a great motivator. Have them answer three consecutive questions you ask them with a definite "Yes" and the sale is done, if they have the actual "yes power" to buy. This has an interesting resemblance to a lion hunt, doesn't it?

Disclaimer: If the customer discovers you've betrayed their trust, unless they're a true believer and will ignore any evidence contrary to the salesperson's integrity, the rapport will be irreparably broken. And they'll tell all their friends

Choosing to be knowledgeable about hypnosis helps one guard the subconscious from unwanted suggestions because you'll recognize a suspect sales pitch. Which is not to say you won't buy anything, but you'll buy it based on your independent decision-making process and will be fairly resistant to the pressure of closers.

Enough with subconscious self-defense. Let's move on to relaxation techniques. Dr. Benson's path is heavily influenced by Transcendental Meditation (TM) as taught by Maharishi Mahesh Yogi, a simple, natural mental technique practiced with the eyes closed while sitting comfortably. The challenge with the relaxation response, Dr. Benson concludes, is that it requires time to set aside and a conscious effort to evoke it, while the fight-or-flight response is automatic. The inference is that one must practice meditation relaxation techniques faithfully in 10-to-20-minute sessions twice a day, so that you can consciously and immediately go into relaxation mode instead of stress mode.

Dr. Selye's foundation has evolved into offering corporate organizational training for using evidence-based stress reduction techniques to enhance profitability. This is way above my pay grade, so I'll stay with what I know about, which is breath, mantras, imagery, and progressive relaxation.

The organization that Jess Stearn, a best-selling author on the occult who came to believe the theories he wrote about, was called Mind Dynamics (which stopped operating around 1973). It was a forebearer of much of the Human Potential Movement, which arose out of the counterculture of the 1960s and formed around the concept of an extraordinary potential that its advocates believed to lie largely untapped in all people. Its teachings were promoted by such motivational training companies as Erhard Seminars Training, or EST, founded by Werner Erhard; Lifespring; and Landmark, some of whose theories have found their way into the culture of corporate leadership training. Everything old is new again.

I've already provided an entire chapter devoted to breathing, so I'll try not to be redundant. Meditation breathing is diaphragmatic breathing, with your attention focused on a point of concentration or not. TM breathing discourages concentration and instead has you just be aware of each breath in and out. Alternate nostril breathing is a yoga technique which requires physical action beyond just breathing, so not useful for meditation. The 4-7-8 method will relax and enable you to achieve calm diaphragmatic breathing for good meditation. There are other helpful breathing exercises, for example, "The Full Breath" technique used for Heart Rhythm Meditation. It sounds terrific, but I'll leave it to you to explore that more fully on your own.

Mantras deserve more explanation, but this will be a brief note because the subject matter is too extensive for this work. Traditionally, mantras were part of yoga meditation and were a secret, because the advice was given only to those who had been chosen by the teacher.

These teachings were highly personalized intonations given one-on-one from teacher to student. A mantra is now considered a word, a sound, or even a phrase or sentence used to focus or center an individual or a group. No teacher has gifted me a personal mantra. I can't pronounce Sanskrit very well, anyway. I do believe the vibration of intoning "Om" or "Aum" or "I AM" is beneficial, but I'm not exactly sure why. It may be that "Om" is interchangeable with "Aum," which is very close to the metaphysical Biblical "I AM," which may explain why most of the mantras I know of I consider to be affirmations. If they work for you, use them. I use them occasionally, but I'm able to meditate without them. To keep me from thinking too much, I enjoy silently repeating "Love" as a mantra when I'm on my daily walks. It's a better method of focused concentration than trying to simultaneously walk and chew gum. That's all for now.

Imagery involves the imagination and memory. We have this marvelous ability to conjure up in our mind's eye images that represent beautiful people, places, and things that bring up feelings of loving, belonging, and safety. The opposite is also true, but that's stressful and we're going to ignore the other side of the coin right now and stay positive. Out of sight, out of mind. It is a worthwhile activity to create a perfect "happy place" so that we can go back there whenever we want. I have a variety of places to go, depending on what's stimulating me to escape perceived reality at the time. Sometimes it's a cool forest glade, and sometimes a hammock between two palm trees on a beach in the tropics is involved. Often it's the memory of holding my children for the first time, or a grandson at two years old, climbing into my lap unbidden and saying "I love you, Oma" spontaneously. It's always good to infuse love into a meditation process to make it more pleasurable. As a matter of fact, in 2009, Dr. Eva Selhub, who was a senior physician at the Benson-Henry Institute for Mind Body Medicine and a clinical instructor of medicine at Harvard Medical School, published a book titled *The Love Response* which elaborated on Dr. Benson's relaxation response, a helpful way to turn off the fight-or-flight response and bring the body back to pre-stress levels.

Guided imagery is also used in self-hypnosis as a means to deepen the state of relaxation. Guided imagery involves mentally experiencing objects or people using the memory of your five senses. An example would be to visualize an apple. Make it the most perfect red apple you can imagine. Notice the shape and size of the apple and where the stem is inserted and how the bottom of the apple looks. Notice the curvature of the apple. Now that you have the picture of the apple in your mind, take a comfortable, easy bite out of it. Feel the tension of your teeth against the skin as it breaks. Hear the crisp sound the act of biting into the apple makes. Notice the difference in the texture as you bite through the skin into the cool flesh inside. Inhale the aroma, as this is the most aromatic apple you have ever experienced. Taste the sweet apple juice as you chew and feel it ever so slightly running out of the corners of your mouth. Hear the sound you make while chewing this juicy, fragrant, delicious red apple. Continue to enjoy experiencing the gift of this apple in perfect contentment.

Did you get into it? Enjoyable, yes? The distraction of full-immersion imagination tends to relieve tension and anxiety.

Progressive muscle relaxation is a technique where major muscle groups of the body are intentionally tensed and then relaxed, so that the individual can feel the difference. Muscle tension is an unconscious physical response to stress. Once you recognize muscle tension, you give your body the suggestion to relax it. Conscious breathing should relax your body, but you need to check that your shoulders are down, your teeth aren't clenched, you're not making fists, and you are in a comfortable body position for that exercise. Suggesting that your body relax completely from the top of your head to the tips of your toes is a step in self-hypnosis, following a deep cleansing breath and a course of four square breathing cycles. On the last exhalation of the cycle, breathe out completely, close your eyes, and resume breathing normally in and out through your nose, giving yourself the suggestion to "relax totally and completely now." As you breathe, repeat the suggestion to "relax now" a couple more times.

If you have no experience with being hypnotized or with meditation, self-induction to hypnotize yourself is often helped by using an object to focus on, such as in Lamaze childbirth training. Any object will do. After you have become successful at the practice, you won't need to use eye fixation. Soft background music is helpful—I suggest something with 4/4 time or common time that's on a loop so there won't be any disruptive breaks in the music. By the way, it was discovered back in the day that common time is the meter to put your brain in alpha waves and make learning easier. Relaxation techniques can also put your brain into alpha, so it's a synergistic pairing.

Just sitting or lying in a comfortable position, using a focal point, deep breathing for a cycle, closing your eyes, and repeating a word or phrase like "relax now" three times while allowing your muscles to relax as you belly breathe normally will put you into a state of light hypnosis. Don't try when doing this—just let go. The more you practice, the easier it will become to relax. I do not mean this chapter to be an in-depth tutorial on hypnosis; there are plenty of other authoritative sources. I just wanted to provide a brief, pleasurable, easy way to prove to you that you can do it when you want to and give you a basis from which to expand, if you wish.

A delightful side effect of relaxation is that it makes us happy, because we are free of conscious cares. Although we are aware of our physical surroundings, we are unconcerned. It is like the state you're in when you're dropping off to sleep and can hear a clock ticking, but you are undisturbed by it. If the sound was important, you'd wake up, but it's not, so you choose to ignore it. Your attention is focused inward rather than outward.

So, to recap, these four techniques: Imagination can cause worry and stress, but it also provides the antidote by providing a pathway to mindfulness and relaxation. Paradoxically, mindfulness involves not thinking and relaxation requires focused concentration. You have a basic overview map. Set your own course.

There are two good ways to get immediate relief from stress. One is deep relaxation. I touched on exercises for relaxation. The other is laughter. Just like we can practice relaxation techniques until the reaction is automatic to the stimulus of stress, so can we practice until we develop a laughter response. This comes about by keeping the slings and arrows of outrageous fortune in perspective and truly appreciating our great fortune in being alive.

It's sometimes a hard sell to the health-care establishment that a non-pharmaceutical agent can act like a miracle drug—and it's free, to boot. Laughter can be the equivalent of a self-administered placebo. Several placebo effect studies over the last decade on the treatment of migraine headaches found that a placebo (dummy pill) was considered to be 50% as effective as pain medication. Clinical studies demonstrated placebos administered for pain control can trigger the natural pharmacy in your brain to release endogenic opioids (natural pain-relieving chemicals). Somehow, by just believing that the pill they give you provides pain relief, your body activates your pain relief system. Pretty cool, huh?

Pain causes tension in the body because it is a warning that something is off-kilter. Pain is a great attention-getter. If you relieve the pain, the body relaxes and attempts to return to homeostasis, or its best baseline. Placebos as therapy seem to be most effective in cases where the underlying health problem is related to stress. Self-care practices can also act as placebos. An important element of self-care is keeping your sense of humor and allowing it to express itself through laughter.

American humor writer Bennett Cerf (1898–1971) is often given credit as the origin of the phrase "Laughter is the best medicine," but the belief behind the metaphor is ancient. The source for the phrase is probably from the Jewish tradition's Proverbs of Solomon, which are in the genre of wisdom literature. The referenced section translates as "A happy heart is good medicine, but low spirits sap one's strength." Similar translations show up in the Christian Bible.

Professional comedians and humorists endorse the phrase as gospel—after all, laughter is their business. In the Star Trek movie *The Wrath of Khan*, the Vulcan character Saavik comments to Admiral Kirk, "Humor. It is a difficult concept. It is not logical." Because laughter is not logical, it disrupts our brain's routine ways of organizing information by introducing something random, giving us the superpower to introduce new concepts into our thought processes and confound our monkey brain. Plus, we can share the joy.

Scientific findings show that laughter is contagious, and that the left side of the brain seems to set up the joke while the right side understands it. Studies have also shown measurable positive physical reactions to humor and laughter that increase immunity, decrease stress hormones, help the respiratory and cardiac systems, and increase pain control. Laughter can be compared to internal jogging. There is a scientifically unproven meme that 1 minute of anger weakens the immune system for 4 to 5 minutes, but 1 minute of laughter boosts the immune system for 24 hours. Doesn't it seem that laughter is better for you than anger?

Humor and laughter are not the same, of course. Laughter is sometimes the response to humor. There are jokes that bring up things that are out of place in the context that bring on a laugh to relieve the tension of that situation, as well as stories about human nature that highlight our common ability to make mistakes where laughter can lighten the mood or change how we look at things. Although they don't seem to be funny, the most popular topics for humor are sex, religion, and death.

It is the physical act of laughing that provides physical benefits, not the subject matter that brought out the belly laugh. Laughter can be naturally triggered by humor or artificially caused by conscious laughter-inducing behavior. It's beneficial either way. Case in point, laughing yoga. And not to be overlooked, those stalwarts of novelty shops' inventory, the whoopee cushion (along with its remote-controlled, hidden recorded version) and the Laugh Bag, a battery powered individually sized recording of canned laughter in a bag (duh), a la comedy show audience reaction on demand. No judgment—I'm all for whatever will make us laugh.

Writer and philosopher G. K. Chesterton is quoted as saying, "Life is serious all the time, but living cannot be. You may have all the solemnity that you wish in choosing your neckties, but in anything important, such as death, sex, and religion, you must have mirth or you will have madness."

Humor and laughter help us cope during times of crisis. What makes you laugh? Watching silly animal antics on YouTube? Watching comedy performances on TV or the internet? Reading, or being read to out loud from humorous books or joke collections? Talking to friends about your humorous reactions to observations about human nature? Let's face it, people's behavior can be funny—ours included—and we're allowed to laugh, even in times of disaster.

My mother introduced me to various forms of humor, because it was her best defense in life and she wanted to pass on that coping mechanism. She pointed out the humor in dicey situations so that I would make a habit of noticing it and be amused to the point of laughter, rather than becoming angry or sad. It is preferable to laugh and feel empowered than to feel pissed off and helpless.

She also shared *Reader's Digest* magazine with me at a young age, which contained several sections of humor material. I have a collection of their stories in book form, as well as other joke books and humor collections I read until I laugh out loud, when the occasion calls for getting out of a vortex of seriousness.

Mark Twain wrote, "The human race has only one really effective weapon, and that is laughter." You can't hate your neighbor when you're laughing with them. A pioneer in the therapeutic use of laughter, the late Dr. William F. Fry, Jr., a psychiatrist at Stanford University, wrote that the United States has raised "war generations" that have adopted direct violent actions as their response to frustration and stress because that is their primary learned coping mechanism. Humor offers a creative alternative to violence, lifting humanity up above the results of violence and warfare.

Laughter is a physical reaction to humor that is followed by a relaxation response. Two physical stress related behaviors—cigarette smoking and overeating—are not possible to do while laughing. I had the good fortune of meeting the late Norman Cousins when he, Alan Funt (the creator of *Candid Camera* in the 1940s, still on YouTube), and a psycho-neuroimmunologist whose name escapes me gave a small group presentation to nurses in the late 1980s on clinically demonstrated positive physical effects of laughter.

Norman wrote a bestselling book about the therapeutic value of laughter in his recovery from an intractable disease, *Anatomy of an Illness as Perceived by the Patient: Reflections on Healing and Regeneration*. He sequestered himself in a hotel room with videos that made him laugh out loud, took copious quantities of vitamin C, and refused to accept doctors' opinions that what he had was incurable. Norman reported getting hours of healing sleep after as little as 10 minutes of belly laughs. He benefited greatly from what amounted to self-administered placebos. I think this would be better as, while there were some clinical theories about vitamin C, Norman had a holistic approach. His laughter routine by itself couldn't be solely credited for his recovery. It contributed significantly. Rather than wait until a horrible disease befalls us to see if we can replicate his results, I think that laughter as a preventative measure is important.

French philosopher Voltaire wrote, "The art of medicine consists in amusing the patient while nature cures the disease." Wouldn't it be interesting if physicians were required to take a course in humor in health care? I would recommend Patch Adams (Dr. Hunter Doherty Adams) as their role model.

I have to admit, before I grew that hideous polyp in my stomach, my personal sense of humor was fairly dormant. Which is a strange thing, since I have the daily goal of making at least one person I come into contact with laugh. I seem to have a gift for being able to do that, but I didn't always join in the actual laughter, which is unfortunate. I love to laugh. Now when I catch myself not laughing enough, I stage a personal intervention. I have to give myself permission to have intermittent bouts of happiness and refuse to take my concern about the state of the world's affairs too seriously.

Human life is basically a play with tragic and comedic interpretations for every act. There is a saying that tragedy plus time equals comedy. Happiness comes from the ability to find humor and express it with laughter. Usually, the missing ingredient is the time to put it in perspective. As Will Rogers, a Native American vaudeville performer, actor, and humorous social commentator from the Cherokee tribe, said, "Everything is funny as long as it is happening to somebody else." Imagine seeing yourself as "the somebody else" in a challenging personal situation and notice if your attitude toward it changes. Find humor in the most difficult situations to help you accept and overcome hardship.

Affirmation Examples:

"I choose to laugh at this situation, finding the
humor in this challenging situation."

"Laughter flows easily through me and
I am filled with joy."

"I embrace my healing energy every time
I laugh or smile."

Healing Exercise:

As an exercise to demonstrate the healing power of laughter, I'm going to ask for audience participation. I don't know your personal sense of humor. Imposing one's humor on another risks being offensive, so I'm going to suggest that you start a humor journal and scrapbook and use it.

You can start by writing down humorous memories from your life and then sharing them with family and friends when/if appropriate. You can journal entries of funny things that happened each day or however frequently you'd like. Include scrapbook jokes or cartoons that make you laugh. Stick to constructive and positive humor, avoiding anti-ethnic or put-down humor, because cruel humor is always mean and never funny. List movies, YouTube videos, books, etc., that you can turn to for laughter when you're in need of it. I'm a big fan of the Pink Panther movie series with Peter Sellers (or the Steve Martin remake) and anything Monty Python, which reveals my advanced age. The Monty Python troupe is well into their 70s now and still irreverent and silly. They have been the rock stars of comedy for over a half century, demonstrating what Irish writer Arland Ussher observed: "Humor is the sense of the absurd which is despair refusing to take itself seriously." You might buy a whoopee cushion or a Laugh Bag. When you turn your attention to humor and laughter, your attitude will reflect that focus.

Follow-Up Thoughts:

Laughter is universal, international, and timeless. A brief history of laughter: The oldest known joke is on a Sumerian cuneiform tablet from 3100–2900 B.C. (It's a fart joke.) There is humor in the ancient Vedas from India, and ancient Chinese jokes are much like contemporary Western humor, using a lot of puns. Ancient Greek physicians prescribed visiting the Hall of Comedians for their patients. African proverbs and riddles have an undercurrent of humor. Early Native American tribes had clowns who got the crowd laughing prior to some ceremonies, because laughter was considered a gift from the spirits and helped in opening the people up to what the spirits wanted them to learn.

Today there are laughter clubs throughout the world because the practice has documented health benefits. Laughing yoga began around 1995 to encourage deep breathing and laughter. Forced laughter on exhale sounds fake at first, but it's so silly that others join in with authentic laughter and soon all are enjoying the feelings of well-being laughter provides. Factoid: The first Sunday in May is World

Laughter Day. Who knew? I like that a day is officially dedicated to laughter, but we have the choice to dedicate a bit of every day to laughter. Laugh and be happy. The world will be a better place for it.

"If you do not change direction,
you may end up where you are heading."

—LAO TZU

CHAPTER SEVEN
Changing

Taking Love-Based Responsibility for
Choosing to Set a More Restorative Course

CHANGE IS INEVITABLE, so being flexible is important. We can control our reaction to unexpected changes, as well as our behavior to initiate our own changes. But lasting change is a challenge. We need to be gentle with ourselves and not let perfect get in the way of good. We need to breathe deeply, fill ourselves with feelings of unconditional love, and make ourselves laugh despite whatever perceived blocks to our happiness appear.

My late brother, Michael, a fine chiropractor, used to lament about his patients' resistance to compliance with his treatment plans. His favorite saying was, "No change will occur until the pain of change is less than the pain of the status quo."

My preferred approach to life is to proceed from the premise that our lives are all a story, and since our lives are composed of our stories, we're free to embellish and edit them anyway we want. Some people resist change because it would appear to be an admission that they were wrong, and nobody likes to be wrong. Some people embrace change, I guess, because they're up for new adventures and easily bored. I wouldn't know. I'm not a natural fan of change, but I'm coming to accept it. I'm a fan of safety, and the results of change are unknown and therefore risky. However, even someone as risk-averse as me can benefit from the realization that change is going to occur, whether we welcome it or not. I'm thinking that it's better to be the agent of change in our own lives than to only be reactive to the changes that others thrust into our lives. We can use that glorious double-edged sword of free will and choose change.

Choice comes from the inside and chance comes from the outside. To paraphrase Carl Jung, until we make the unconscious conscious, we will call what happens in our lives fate. Our inside choices can influence the actions of the outside world by reaction, or so I believe based on my life experience. Choice is becoming more proactive in your life. And choice infers change. My experience is that our judgment of life experiences as good or bad changes with hindsight and reflection. We have the choice to change how we interpret our experiences and change our perception of our lives. When we choose to change our thinking, we choose to change our life.

History, long considered to be an objective record of what happened, is actually fluid and changeable based on the chronicler's interpretation of the results of the events. History is constantly being rewritten as evolving facts are discovered and old misinterpretations are discarded. The story of our lives can be changed by reframing situations considering new evidence. There's an old saying that something happened, we made up a story about it, and lived our lives as if the story was true. Well, maybe it was true for us for a while, but we could not have known all the contributory conditions. Regardless, it's our story, and we can change it based on our current circumstances.

Since we don't live in a vacuum, how do we make permanent, positive personal changes when life's circumstances are constantly changing due to the choices others made without consulting us? Well, perhaps we should try embracing the wisdom of uncertainty and letting go of the illusion of control, especially regarding anything outside ourselves.

Relieve yourself of the uselessness of worry and stress. Unpredictable stuff is going to happen whether or not we worry about it. We prepare as best we can with the information we have, and then go with the flow. Take back your power and the whole game will change.

Change is good.

Affirmation Examples:

"I make healthy choices that create infinite amounts of choices for my highest good."

"I allow my independence to flow and become more empowered."

"I am flexible and free to choose peace, joy, and happiness."

Healing Exercise:

Center yourself. Breathe slowly and deeply, in and out, until you feel calm and collected. Then write down a list of potential life changes. Next, mark which ones you want to initiate and those that are being called for by others. Now prioritize. Are any of the changes literally a matter of life or death? Rewrite the list from the most important life changes to the least. Next, list changes that have been thrust upon you by circumstances beyond your control. These usually involve a loss of some sort. Turn that coin over to see what the positive side reveals. There is always more than one side to a loss.

There will always be an alternative, but it takes time to put it in perspective. Be gentle with yourself and accept the unanticipated, for this pain will help you tap depths of courage that you didn't recognize before. You will rediscover your light and power, and that energy will assist you in the next changes on the list, which are changes you purely want. Set your course, be kind to yourself, and proceed.

If you feel others are pushing unnecessary changes on you that you don't want or need, blow them off. They need to remember to let you live your own life. Sacred selfishness, remember?

Change boils down to exercising self-responsibility. We are not victims. We have the ability to change our minds about preconceived ideas regarding our life circumstances. If you are in a hurry, slow down. If you are worried, stop. Take time to breathe, be still, and listen to the still small voice within. Make peace with uncertainty. Remember, it's OK not to know everything. You are enough. You are always doing your best in the existing circumstances. Celebrate the joys of your imperfection, since it's inherent in human nature and a potential source of laughter. You are making progress, whether you see it now or not. And you've come all this way by deciding to make changes.

If you're not having a pleasant experience, stop and recognize your reaction and behavior. Let go of it, breathe into your belly, relaxing into the ever-present energy of love, and laugh as though this situation is beyond absurd and silly. Lock this preferred experience into your memory to use as a response in the future. Recognize, relax, reframe, and repeat as needed.

So, a current theory is that if you want permanent change in personal behavior, you do it in easy, short, pleasurable steps. In Japan, this method is called kaizen. Kaizen is an action plan based on the philosophy of continuous small improvements.

Now, I know that I profess to be a holistically inclined health coach. However, much of what follows is only mind/body based, coming out of the area of psychology concerned with behavior modification and clinically observed neurological responses to those behaviors. The research is concerned with forming new habits by making a conscious decision to change and then basically rewiring your brain for the new habits.

The spiritual component would be self-recognition that the behaviors you choose to change are out of line with your personal version of the Big Picture and could use realignment. Body informs mind and mind informs body, but the mind can be either lowercase or uppercase "M," as in physical brain mind or spiritual soul Mind. Use whatever interpretation suits you.

The physical brain is resistant to change because the habits it encourages have been established as providing pleasure or safety. Habits are focused on immediate well-being and not long-term benefit. A habit is an autopilot system. Once ingrained it doesn't require attention as long as it's being rewarded. The differentiation is that good habits have long-term benefits and bad ones do not.

Based on neurological research, permanent behavior changes for dropping a bad habit require a lifelong commitment to the change because neural pathways in the brain are permanent. We overlay the new habit pattern over the old one, realizing the old one will always be lurking underneath and so we must be vigilant. We must convince our unconscious mind that the rewards of a good habit are better than those of a bad habit. We do this by reframing and changing undesired habitual thoughts. We make a conscious decision to choose which habit—the new or the old—to express.

The good news is that the brain is only interested in the next 10 minutes. According to John Medina, a molecular biologist at the University of Washington, you have 9 minutes and 59 seconds to keep your audience's attention. After that, you have to take active steps to keep them engaged. Despite the growth of social media and bite-sized nuggets of content, the 10-minute rule seems to remain intact. It also applies around the world. If we can delay reinforcing the undesired behavior for 10 minutes, the urge will go away. To reinforce a new habit, force yourself to repeat something until you don't have to force it anymore. Repetition strengthens the new pathway.

A quick word about the difference between habits and addiction. An addiction always involves a nonpositive habit, but a habit is not necessarily an addiction. Getting up at the same time every day is a habit. Smoking a cigarette the minute you wake up is an addiction. Addiction is like a bad habit on steroids, the steroids being a psychological component which may or may not be caused by a change in brain chemistry triggered by the bad habit. Addiction is an overwhelming compulsion to engage in damaging behavior in spite of harmful consequences. They stimulate the area in the brain associated with rewarding activities needed for survival like eating, having sex, and spending time with friends. Replacing destructive reward-inducing behaviors with positive ones is the goal of rehabilitation.

Here is how I finally quit smoking cigarettes after multiple serious attempts, some of which were successes lasting years. First off, I made the decision that I was doing this for the rest of my life, not just to prove that I could stop anytime I wanted to. This commitment is huge. It shut the door on reconciling with a habit that had been my constant companion since high school. That finality was scary, because there's a part of my reptilian brain that thinks it will die without cigarettes. I started carrying a bottle of water with me all the time, and when I wanted to smoke, I took a sip of water instead. In between sips of water, I took slow, deep breaths, basically air-smoking, repeating the mantra "I am a happy, healthy nonsmoker now and for the rest of my life." This was to further reinforce my new good habit of drinking water and deep breathing instead of smoking. The first three days were the toughest while the nicotine got out of my system, and not having a cigarette was a constant conscious choice for at least a month. There is a thing called the 21-Day Habit Theory, which suggests that any behavior practiced for 21 days consecutively will stick. But you know what? Any new behavior practiced every day for the rest of your life will stick, and you can take that to the bank.

Acknowledge and accept the old pathway is still there. The reptilian brain can exercise its mistaken survival/pleasure drive decades after the addictive behavior has ceased and tempt someone into trying it again, just this once. This usually occurs when we're hanging around people who are using the substance and appearing to have fun, and we want to be a part of it. In extreme cases, relapses into rapidly lethal habits can kill former opioid users and alcoholics. I haven't had a cigarette in nearly 40 years, but every once in a while, it still looks like a pleasurable thing to do, and I briefly miss it. Recognize, relax, reframe, refrain, repeat. The craving will only last a few minutes. Walk away—briskly. I call that "taking a lap."

Withdraw yourself from temptation.

The best way to learn a new desired habit is to copy someone who has successfully achieved your goal. Efforts to quit or modify a habit will fail if they only address depriving yourself of something. It's absolutely necessary to replace one for one. You are not going to be able to permanently replace something perceived as pleasure with the pain of deprivation.

Follow-Up Thoughts:

Take little steps that are easy and fun. Pay attention to the little steps rather than the huge goal. Trust you'll get there, step by step. New habits are established in their own unique-to-you time frame. We may never feel "ready to change," so take whatever small steps seem possible right now and repeat the next hour, the next day, and the day after that. Let go of trying and just do it. When asked how to eat an elephant, a wise person replied, "One bite at a time." Same premise, even if the literal meaning makes me gag.

So, change can be good and good changes can be permanent, which is comforting because change is inevitable. We're inundated with messages that we should change to keep up with the progress of our culture, but since we are the captain of our ship, we have the ability to choose changes that serve our purposes, not someone else's.

"Knowledge is of no value
unless you put it into practice."

—ANTON CHEKHOV

CHAPTER EIGHT

Practice, Practice, Practice

Being Proactive in Reinforcing Radical Loving Self-Care Practices

I FIND IT EASY TO CHANT "Thank you" to whom it may concern every morning upon awakening. I still don't always realize that I'm deserving of my undying (pun intended) gratitude, too. Keeping up the health and well-being practices that I used to overcome a potentially disastrous malady has been an ongoing challenge since I was given an all-clear by the surgeon. During the prolonged first wave of the COVID-19 pandemic with all its attendant social upheaval, the news distracted me a tad from my stated purpose of loving the world back to health by first loving myself and sharing those practices with others of similar interest.

In early March 2020, my husband had symptoms consistent with those of being infected with the virus. He was very sick for three weeks with a cough, fever, shortness of breath, headache, muscle aches, fatigue—well you get the picture. By phone, one of his physicians told him to stay home because medicine had nothing to offer him at that point—no testing to confirm or deny it was indeed the novel coronavirus, nor any definitive treatment if it was—and venturing out was a bad idea for himself and others.

The doctor told him he would be better at home getting one-on-one nursing care from his RN wife, who would know if and when to call 911. I did energy work with myself and with him, but I also observed all the safety precautions possible, gave us supplements, and used all the practices I've shared in this book. My only symptoms were an awful headache, swollen glands, and a sore throat for about a week. As an aside, both of us had flu vaccines and pneumonia vaccines, we have HEPA-filter air purifiers in the most used rooms in our apartment, and my husband has a CPAP. When it was deemed safe enough to have labs, we had antibody testing in mid-June, and the results for both of us were no detectable antibodies. Our physician told us the test was inconclusive about if we'd had it, because even if we did, the antibodies could be gone in three months. So, we behaved as if we already had it and as though we had never had it, because nobody knew for sure.

When I was young, I could have an active strep throat infection and not have any symptoms but be able to infect others, so I dealt with this using the same mindset. Stay home unless the trip is necessary, wear a mask if going out, avoid close contact with others not in my household, wash my hands often, and disinfect common surfaces. So far, so good.

My affirmation was that I'm immune, but I'll be vaccinated. I continued to follow behavioral advice to be a good example to others who may not share my worldview and who also may not have any immunity to an invisible agent of infection I may be carrying. I was not acting out of fear; I was acting with cooperative consideration. I know from my life experiences that my mindset for health, which is holistic, works for me, so it would seem it could benefit others because I'm not that unusual. I am normal, only more so.

What I'm getting to in a roundabout way is that the daily practice of the exercises in this book may help people who would enjoy having some proactive health behaviors that may enrich their life experience, because they helped me. So, if a practice resonates with you, integrate it into your life and notice the positive changes. Pay attention to yourself. You're worth your time and effort.

This is not a comprehensive collection of all the radical loving self-care activities in the known world. Maybe this book will just prompt you to seek some seemingly unrelated subject or practice that enhances your life. It's all good.

I had to limit what I shared in this book so I could finish it. Certainly, all the subjects warrant elaboration. Personally, I'm someone who likes compilations, condensed versions, and shortcuts. The best part of my offering as I see it is that the techniques don't really require a great deal of effort beyond setting your personal compass for your own North Star and venturing forth.

So, love and respect yourself, breathe deeply, laugh and relax, make the changes you want, forgive with gratitude, eat clean, move, sleep, and connect with fellow humans as best you can. There you have it. My path back to health in one sentence. I have enjoyed sharing my journey with you and hope you have gained something from the experience.

Affirmation Examples:

"I control my mind and choose to remain calm."

"The peace in my heart creates ripples throughout my life and those around me."

"I live each day with radiant joy and gratitude."

Healing Exercise:

Here are some suggestions to jump-start new habits for daily healing practices that work for me:

• Keep your journal and a pencil at your bedside. That way you can write down your first thoughts and/or dream images when you awaken.

• Lay in your bed for a few minutes when you wake up, relax, and invite life-force energy to infuse every cell in your body for your highest good.

- As you arise, sit on the edge of your bed and greet the new day with a few deep breaths, setting the tone with a little prayer: *May this day bring peace, forgiveness, and love. Thank you!*

- Recite quietly to yourself a form of grace before eating and drinking, thanking the source of the nourishment and the hands that brought it to you.

- Find something positive that consistently makes you laugh and allow yourself to laugh every day.

- Schedule regular breaks during the day to move your body and breathe deeply.

- Memorize/repeat silent affirmations that counter stress.

Follow-Up Thoughts:

Radical loving self-care is about being comfortable in service to yourself before you offer service to another. The Earth was not created to be a slave planet. Do not give away your personal power. Maintain your sovereignty. We are the masters of our own lives, and we are our own servants first. When we are secure in our own self-mastery journey, we can offer loving help to others without being subservient. We can be in cooperation for the greater good rather than competition. And the world will be a better place.

Afterword

There is an organization, the Institute of Noetic Sciences, that published *Spontaneous Remission: An Annotated Bibliography* in 1993. No standard reference had been created on that subject prior to that. They provided a definition of spontaneous remission:

> "The disappearance, complete or incomplete, of a disease or cancer without medical treatment or treatment that is considered inadequate to produce the resulting disappearance of disease symptoms or tumor."

Please notice that this definition does not mean "instantaneous" healing. It basically covers confirmed cases when a patient's improvement cannot be attributed to Western allopathic medical treatments.

Remission also does not mean regression. Regression is a term used to describe a solid tumor or mass getting smaller or disappearing without any treatment or a treatment that is not adequate to cause this. Spontaneous regression also describes a disease that is not considered cured, where the regression may or may not be complete or permanent.

The research in *Spontaneous Remission: An Annotated Bibliography* cataloged medically reported cases of spontaneous remission all over the world, using more than 800 journals in 20 different languages. That information alone should provide adequate validation for the phenomena. When there is enough evidence presented by independent credible sources, I think it's acceptable as reality. One white crow is enough proof that all crows are not black. Spontaneous remission happens. And if others can do it, it follows that so can we.

Other writers elaborated on this information and, through an interview process, came up with a consensus of what the successful patients changed in their lives. Most of these patients had been diagnosed with cancer. These changes included cleaning up their diet; taking vitamins and supplements to boost their immune system; interacting with a spiritual community; filling themselves with love, joy, and happiness; letting go of unproductive emotions like fear, anger, and resentment; using their powerful inner knowing to guide their treatment options; and having strong reasons to live.

Kelly A. Turner, PhD, in her book *Radical Remission: Surviving Cancer Against All Odds*, defined three factors as the foundation of successfully positively changing one's health status. They are having a strong reason to live, taking personal control of your health, and accepting social support (which includes the unconditional love of pets, by the way).

My path to healing was guided primarily by spiritual and psychological factors: hypnosis, altered states of consciousness (e.g. meditation and Reiki), placebos, and the group support of my social support and spiritual community that surrounded me with strength once I made the necessary internal changes. Running in the background was my understanding of the Twelve Steps. Before I was diagnosed, I was pretty self-satisfied about my good health, being an RN holistic health coach and wanting to teach by example.

Humility has been a gentle yet persistent teacher for me. I asked for the prayers of my spiritual community, joined a small daily prayer group, and asked to be put on prayer lists when anyone offered. This was fairly uncharacteristic for me. Afterwards, I was told that people I'd never met were praying for me; friends had asked on my behalf, as they were concerned about my health even though I hadn't told them my diagnosis. I'm convinced that the energy of those healing intentions gave me beneficial effects. I didn't walk my healing path alone. Gratitude for that unconditional love is the primary motivation for writing this book.

When I was employed as a nurse and health coach, I was aware of information about nontraditional therapies and shared what I could on a one-on-one basis with my clients-patients. As a corporate health-care employee, I often had to tiptoe between different therapies described in what was once termed by the National Institutes of Health as the National Center for Complementary and Alternative Medicine, and is now the National Center for Complementary and Integrative Medicine as of December 2014.

There is also a separate Office of Cancer Complementary and Alternative Medicine in the National Cancer Institute. The American medical establishment is historically territorial in approving treatment plans for diseases and injuries. Interestingly, other countries with full access to Western medicine have not discarded the therapies that healed prior to the current scientific era. There was no reason to fix something that wasn't broken.

Anyway, I realized that I was doling out holistic healthcare advice in a very piecemeal fashion on an as needed basis. It's such a huge, specialized database, and there didn't seem to be any handy, easy-to-use primer that I could find that people could use as a quick reference to get well and stay well. For millennia, healing was connected to religion and philosophy; then, just in the last couple hundred years, Western civilization began emphasizing treating the body like a machine instead of like a super complicated material expression of consciousness.

I discovered that once I retired from active nursing, without the constant reminders of wellness practices that I shared with my clients, I stopped mindfully practicing a lot of what I had preached. Once I was out of an actively health-promoting environment, I found myself passively absorbing and imitating the unhealthy behaviors of those I was around. Without the motivation to be a good example for my children and my clients, I got lazy. Maintenance can be a chore, and it takes a bit of effort to maintain a healthy lifestyle. Good habits need to be reinforced and bad habits need to be recognized and changed, and I've found it depends on how I feel when I wake up each day. It's not that mindful choices will allow our bodies to live forever. It's just that I'd like to be as pain-free and comfortable as possible from Point A to Point B.

And this discussion brings us back to the Big Picture, which is always playing in the background. In the Big Picture, to live on Earth fully, we need to have death in our viewfinder, because our bodies start on their march toward inevitable physical death the moment we're born. Not to dwell on it, but just be aware. Death is not the opposite of life; life is eternal and has no opposite. Birth and death are the beginning and the end only in the physical realm. They are both observable by our physical senses, and so they are empirical facts. Our birthright is to die. Too heavy? Wait, there's more.

Scholars and laypeople have been studying death for ages, because why not? It's a fascinating process. And the general agreement, based on scientific and experiential research, is that death is nothing to be afraid of. Death is the expansion, not the destruction, of our consciousness.

Love is the invisible force that connects your soul to your body at birth and then separates them at death. What is the purpose of life? To learn by experience how to love unconditionally, starting with loving ourselves.

Love is why we're here, and everything else is an elaborate interactive play to provide opportunities to express love in different circumstances. So, in the Big Picture of your life, spontaneous remission is just one physical benefit of choosing loving, proactive actions. It's making the conscious choice to practice radical self-love that will get you started on your own healing journey.

And That's the Truth.

Appendix

The Parable Of "Good Luck, Bad Luck, Who Knows?"

I'm finding the situation to be a wonderful opportunity to reconnect with myself, and I realize I am extraordinarily fortunate in that regard. This book is my way of paying it forward. If even one person finds one thing in my experience that makes their path easier, I will have accomplished what I set out to do.

This folktale has a few variations and is sometimes called the Chinese farmer story or the Taoist "Good Luck, Bad Luck, Who Knows?" story, as its earliest origins can be found in the *Tao Te Ching* by Lao Tzu.

A righteous man lived near the border of barbarian territory and farmed his land with his son using his one horse. They used the horse to plow the fields, sow the seeds, and take their goods to the market. One day for no reason, the horse ran off. The neighbors felt sorry for him, saying, "This is such bad luck." But the man responded, "Good luck. Bad luck. Who knows?"

Some time later, the horse returned with a group of wild horses, which the man and his son corralled. The villagers then congratulated him on his good luck. Again, he said,

"Good luck. Bad luck. Who knows?"

The son set about training the wild horses and fell and broke his leg. Now the son would be unable to help his father, who would have to do all the work by himself. Everyone felt sorry for him again. The man replied, "Good luck. Bad luck. Who knows?"

A few days later the emperor's army came into the village and took the able-bodied sons away to fight in a war against the barbarians. The man's son would not be of use with his broken leg, so he was left behind. The villagers commented on the man's good luck that his son was spared. The wise man just said, "Good luck. Bad luck. Who knows?"

So, bad luck brings good luck and good luck brings bad luck. This happens without end, and nobody can predict it.

There are Western parallels to this story in proverbs like "Every cloud has a silver lining," which have a perspective that points to an eventual good outcome. A more neutral one is expressed in a statement from Shakespeare's Hamlet to Rosencrantz: "...for there is nothing either good or bad, but thinking makes it so."

Sound familiar?

The Seven Chakras

The seven chakras are theorized to be the main centers of energy in the etheric body, which is considered to be like the metaphysical twin of our physical body.

The chakras are said to be located parallel to the spine, where they are the main receivers and distributors of vital energy between the physical body and subtle energy fields. They are numbered starting from the base of the spine to the top of the head.

Each chakra reportedly corresponds to a different gland, governs specific parts of the physical body and areas of psychological and spiritual development, and has a color assigned that follows the colors of the rainbow. Balance among the chakras should result in maximum vitality and health. Blockages tied to physical or emotional trauma can show up as a problem in the corresponding body areas. The aim of healing arts such as acupuncture, shiatsu, massage, and energy work is to restore balance and harmony between the individual and the universal life-force energy that is present everywhere.

The Seven Chakras

CHAKRA	GLAND	COLOR	ORGANS	BODY AREA	BEHAVIOR
Crown	Pineal	Violet	Cranium	Head	Spiritual
Brow	Pituitary	Indigo	Ears	Forehead	Intellect
Throat	Thyroid	Sky Blue	Lungs	Arms	Connection
Heart	Thymus	Green	Heart	Chest	Love
Solar Plexus	Pancreas	Yellow	Liver	Stomach	Power Center
Sacral	Gonads	Orange	Genitals	Belly	Sexuality
Root	Adrenals	Red	Kidneys	Legs	Survival

There are plenty of fine examples on the internet and elsewhere.

Suggestions for Further Reading

Here is a recap of the books mentioned in the text, as well as a few I picked out from my many bookcases that might be of interest. They are mostly oldies but goodies and are listed in no particular order.

Anatomy of an Illness as Perceived by the Patient: Reflections on Healing and Regeneration by Norman Cousins

The Relaxation Response by Herbert Benson, MD

The Stress of Life by Hans Selye, MD

The Power of Alpha-Thinking by Jess Stearn

The Love Response by Eva M. Selhub, MD

Spontaneous Remission: An Annotated Bibliography by Brendan O'Regan and Caryle Hirshberg

Radical Remission: Surviving Cancer Against All Odds by Kelly A. Turner, PhD

Mind Over Medicine: Scientific Proof That You Can Heal Yourself by Lissa Rankin, MD

You Can Heal Your Life by Louise L. Hay

The 30-Day Diabetes Miracle by Franklin House, MD, Stuart A. Seale, MD, and Ian Blake Newman

Your Healing Hands: The Polarity Experience by Richard Gordon

Overdiagnosed: Making People Sick in the Pursuit of Health by H. Gilbert Welch, MD, Lisa M. Schwartz MD, and Steven Woloshin, MD

How Doctors Think by Jerome Groopman, MD

The Four Agreements by Don Miguel Ruiz

The Energy Experiments: Science Reveals Our Natural Power to Heal by Gary E. Schwartz, PhD

Any books written by Andrew Weil, MD, or Bernie S. Siegel, MD

About the Author

Mary Joosten Lopata, MA, RN, is a lifelong independent investigator and experiencer of the spirit/mind/body connection as it relates to healing and wellness. Her education in both metaphysics and science has made her simultaneously a believer and an open-minded skeptic. As a consequence, she personally applies to her own life both conventional and alternative and complementary healing techniques she has learned about and shares those that work for her, acknowledging that hers are not the only paths to an individual's optimal health.

Besides being a Registered Nurse for over three decades, Mary is certified as a hypnotherapist and a Reiki Master, and is a member of the American Holistic Nursing Association. She has taught and given health presentations in a variety of settings. She is twice-widowed and resides in Southern California, where she is a hospice volunteer. Her intention is to empower people to rediscover the healer within and integrate that innate knowledge into daily practice, so that healing can take place in spite of dysfunction in the health-care system.

9780875169538